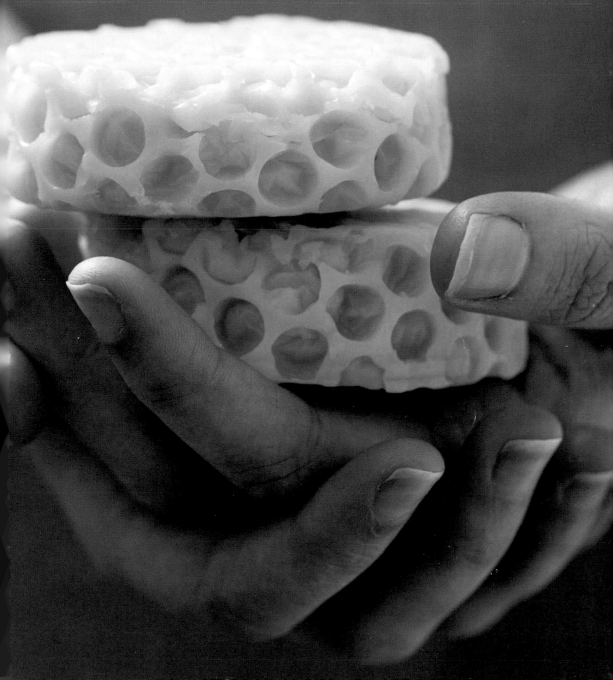

Pure Soapmaking

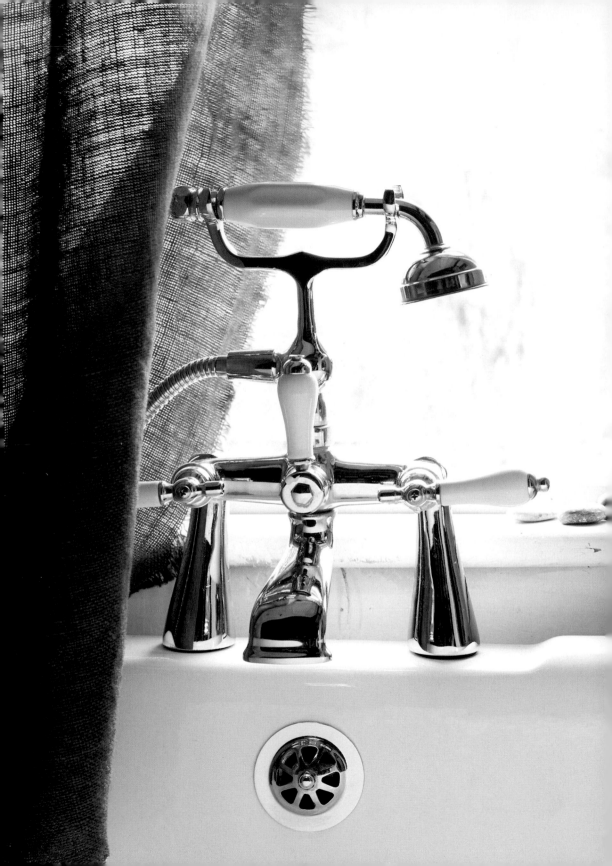

PURE SOAPMAKING

How to Create Nourishing, Natural Skin Care Soaps

ANNE-MARIE FAIOLA

Storey Publishing

*The mission of Storey Publishing is to serve our customers by
publishing practical information that encourages
personal independence in harmony with the environment.*

EDITED BY Lisa Hiley

ART DIRECTION AND BOOK DESIGN BY Michaela Jebb

INDEXED BY Nancy D. Wood

COVER PHOTOGRAPHY BY © Lara Ferroni (author), Mars Vilaubi (back),
and Michaela Jebb (front and spine)

STILL-LIFE PHOTOGRAPHY BY © Tara Donne, **WITH PHOTO STYLING BY** Raina Kattelson: 1–3, 5–8, 11, 18, 42, 54,
68–70, 78, 82, 86, 100–102, 108, 114, 118, 126, 130, 140, 146–148, 158, 162, 166, 178, 182, 186, 190, 198, 204, 210, 218, 224

HOW-TO PHOTOGRAPHY BY © Lara Ferroni: 15, 16, 21–39, 45–50, 58, 60, 64, 72, 73, 76, 77, 80, 81, 84, 85, 88, 89,
92–94, 98, 99, 104–107, 110–112, 115–117, 120, 121, 124, 125, 128, 129, 132–134, 137–139, 142–145, 150–152, 155, 157, 160, 161,
164, 165, 168–171, 174–176, 179–181, 184, 185, 188, 189, 192–196, 199–203, 206–209, 213–217, 220–223, 226–229, 232–236

ADDITIONAL PHOTOGRAPHY BY Mars Vilaubi: 52, 74, 122, 136, 154, and Michaela Jebb: 90, 96, 172, 230

COVER LETTERING BY © Nicolas Fredrickson

Be sure to read all the instructions thoroughly before undertaking any of the projects
in this book and follow all the safety guidelines provided.

Storey Publishing
210 MASS MoCA Way
North Adams, MA 01247
www.storey.com

Printed in China by R.R. Donnelley
10 9 8 7 6 5

LIBRARY OF CONGRESS CATALOGING-IN-PUBLICATION DATA

Names: Faiola, Anne-Marie, author. | Ferroni, Lara,
photographer.
Title: Pure soapmaking : how to create nourishing,
natural skin care soaps / Anne-Marie Faiola, the
Soap Queen ; photography by Lara Ferroni.
Description: North Adams, MA : Storey Publishing,
[2016] | Includes index.
Identifiers: LCCN 2015036737| ISBN 9781612125336
(hardcover : alk. paper) |
ISBN 9781612125343 (ebook)
Subjects: LCSH: Soap.
Classification: LCC TP991 .F279 2016 | DDC 668/.12—
dc23 LC record available at http://lccn.loc
.gov/2015036737

DEDICATION & ACKNOWLEDGMENTS

This book is dedicated to my husband, Chris Renoud. Being married to an entrepreneur is filled with highs and lows, and during the process of writing this book, he took on extra duty at home with our two children and busy household so I could write, soap, edit, and soap some more. My mom and dad have always been there to lend a helping hand throughout my entire entrepreneurial journey and this part of it was no exception. Thank you for letting me bounce ideas off of you and always supporting me.

My team at Bramble Berry is one of the great joys of my life. They do the hard stuff so that I can be creative and focus on all things handmade. I could not do this job without them nor would I want to. A big shout-out to my assistant Caitlin who kept all the recipes, ingredients, colorants, and techniques organized during this writing and testing process.

Finally, thank you to the dedicated group of brand new soapers who tested each recipe in this book to ensure that they would produce amazing bars of soap each and every time.

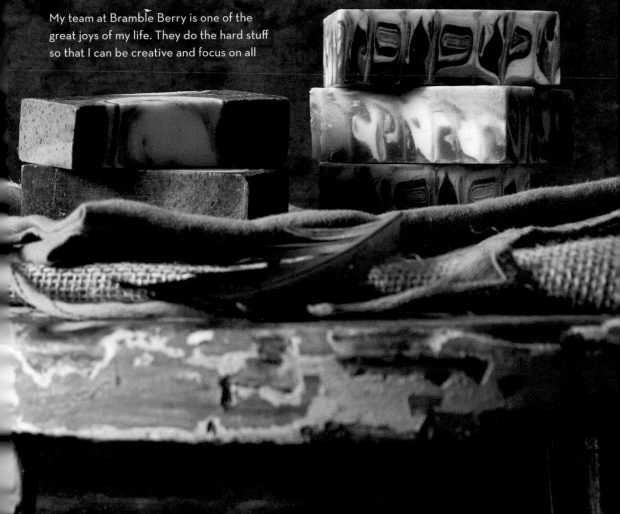

CONTENTS

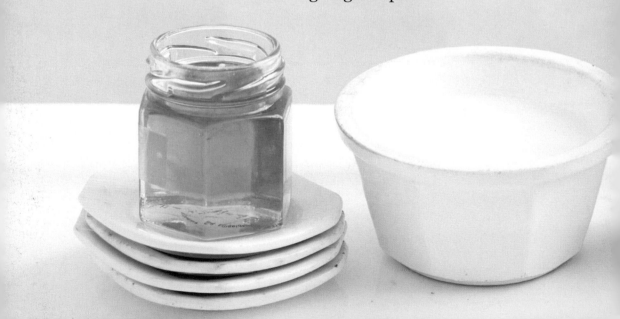

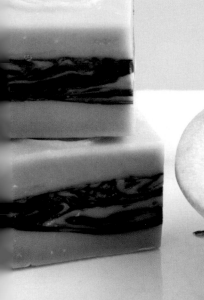

The Beauty of Pure, Handmade Soap

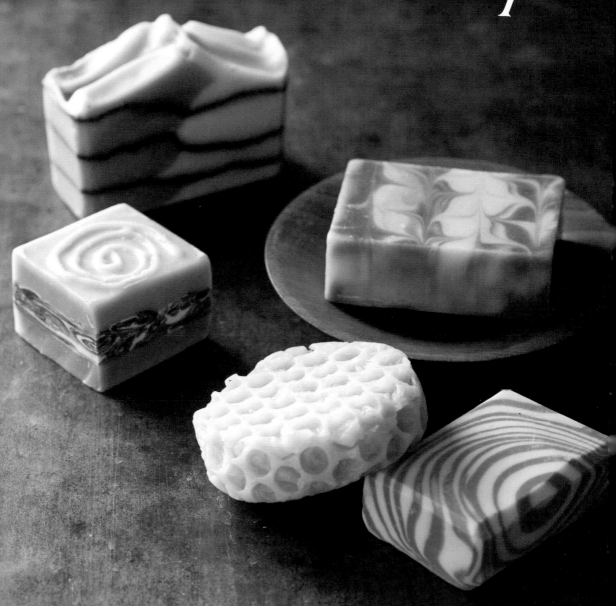

*I*F YOU'VE PICKED up this book, there's a good possibility that you're consciously choosing to reduce synthetic ingredients in your life. Handmade soap lathers and cleanses just as well as commercial soap but doesn't have harsh ingredients, and you can mix and match the ingredients to come up with a soap that is just right for you.

For example, coconut oil is a great cleanser and produces good lather, but used at 100 percent, it can feel drying to some skin. To balance it out, you can combine it with a myriad of other oils that are gentler. Olive oil, for example, is commonly used because skin loves it and it creates a stable, conditioning bar. Avocado oil, sweet almond oil, and rice bran oil contain vitamins and skin-loving fatty acids, and they're cost effective. Castor oil adds extra bubbles. Shea butter and cocoa butter have wonderful moisturizing properties.

With homemade soaps, you control the additives. Ingredients such as coffee grounds and crushed walnut shells add gentle exfoliating power. Oatmeal can provide soothing relief for itchiness. Infused oils provide extra moisturizing and calming properties for difficult skin. Having a pharmacopoeia of custom-made natural soap ingredients means you can create the best product for your skin, using different formulas as needed. This book contains over 30 fully tested recipes for almost every skin type and occasion.

Another reason to make your own soap is that it's an environmentally sound practice. In the past few years, an entire population of soapmakers has picked up the hobby and even entered the business of soapmaking because they were concerned about a variety of issues, including the use of phosphates, which are linked to algae bloom in rivers and streams. Many people also wanted to use ingredients that had not been tested on animals and did not threaten natural resources.

Even using all-natural ingredients can have an environmental impact to consider. For instance, more than half of the recipes in this book are made without palm oil for those who are concerned about the link between palm oil production and the declining ecosystem of orangutans. Orangutans have become the poster child for this issue because nearly 90 percent of their habitat has been destroyed by unsustainable logging in Sumatra and Borneo, placing them on the Endangered Species list. This mass deforestation also affects the habitats of Sumatran tigers, sun bears, clouded leopards, and proboscis monkeys.

Making soap with or without palm oil is a personal choice; while it is possible to soap without palm oil, there is often a trade-off for bar hardness and lather. One option is to purchase certified sustainable palm oil to use in your soapmaking (see What Is Sustainable Palm Oil?, page 40). Knowing the source of your ingredients allows you to make products exactly the way you want them, and make them in good conscience.

Another consideration is the use of genetically modified organisms (GMO) in producing some oils commonly used in cosmetics. There are many non-GMO options for oils and ingredients. You can find many of them at your local health food store or online. Two oils that are commonly GMO are soybean oil and canola oil. If this is a concern for you, look for the "Non-GMO Project Verified" seal, or a suitable counterpart. Additionally, you can check with your vendor if their products are non-GMO.

Avoiding controversial ingredients is possible if you take time to research your ingredients and ask questions of your vendors. You can make soaps that are good for you and the environment.

But most of all, making beautiful soap is just plain fun! Creating something useful and beautiful out of ordinary ingredients brings a thrill like no other. Being able to say, "I made it" is inspiring and delightful. Making your own soap gives you a way to express yourself that is different from painting or sculpting. Soaping offers unlimited opportunities to be creative with colorful designs and beautiful patterns that appeal to any taste. You can make simple, serviceable bars that are lovely in their purity or opt for more complex patterns that create layers or swirls of color. Or go all out with embedded designs that pop from a pretty background. (See Blueberry Embed Round Bars, page 148, or Goat Milk Sunset Burst, page 210.)

Even better, soap is a consumable art form: the more you make, the more you can use, give away, or sell. And once it's used up, you can make more. It is a never-ending creative cycle.

NOTE: The best way to read this book is to review the science parts of the book before diving into soapmaking. If you're just starting out, be sure to read Step-by-Step Cold-Process Soapmaking (starting on page 27). Oatmeal Soap for Babies (page 78) and 100% Castile-Brine Stamped Cube (page 74) are good recipes for beginners to practice with before tackling more intricate designs and techniques.

Happy Soaping!

Anne-Marie

P.S. If you'd like to continue your soapmaking journey, be sure to check out my first book, *Soap Crafting*, or my blog, SoapQueen.com.

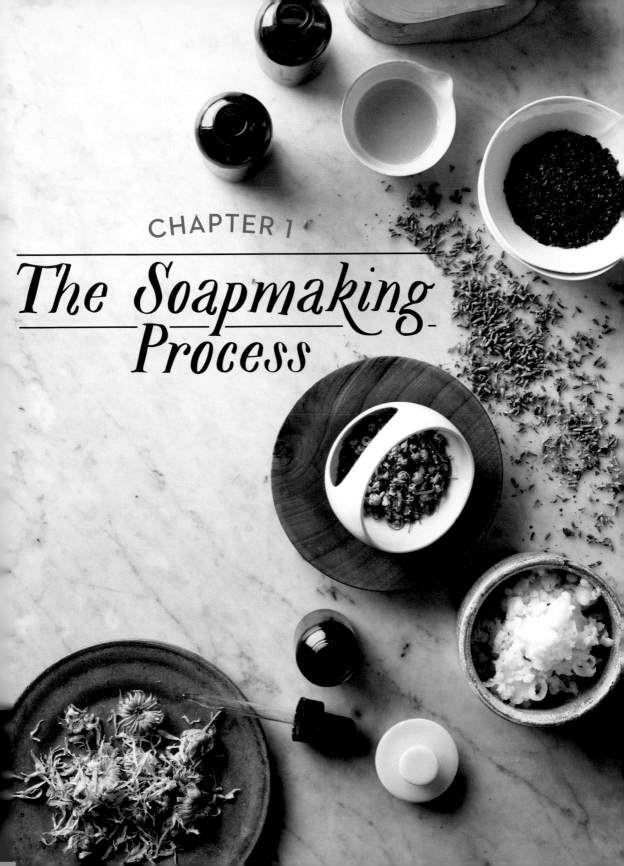

CHAPTER 1

The Soapmaking Process

KNOWING HOW SOAP IS MADE and the science behind it will help you be alert to pitfalls, troubleshoot problems, develop your own recipes, and keep yourself safe during the process. This book primarily focuses on cold-process soapmaking. The term "cold-process" refers to the fact that you don't need to use an outside heat source, such as a stove, during the mixing stage of making soap, although heat is produced during the process. This is because lye mixed with water undergoes an exothermic reaction that can produce temperatures up to 200°F (93°C).

The Science of Soapmaking

The formula for making soap can be written like this:

$$\text{Triglycerides (fatty acids)} + \text{Sodium hydroxide} = \textit{Soap} + \textit{Glycerin}$$

In plain English, oils react with lye to create a solid mass. Oils are made of triglycerides, three fatty acid chains connected with a glycerin molecule. Linoleic acid triglycerides (an essential fatty acid commonly found in soapmaking oils) interact with sodium hydroxide (lye) in a process called saponification. The result of saponification is soap with a small amount of glycerin mixed in.

Sodium hydroxide is typically sold as a powder or flakes. It requires a carrier agent to dissolve it so it can mix with oil. Soapmakers typically dissolve their lye in water, but other liquids may be used.

When lye is added to water, an exothermic (heat-producing) reaction occurs. When substituting other liquids for water, the reaction is often hotter, causing other reactions. For example, lye causes the proteins and sugar in milk to scald, turn yellow, smell badly, and congeal into a thick soup, all of which is normal. Each recipe in this book discusses what to watch out for when soaping with alternative liquids and how to control or minimize problems.

Different oils require different amounts of lye to turn them into soap. The amount of lye needed to turn a specific amount of oil into soap is called the saponification (SAP) value (see What Is the SAP Value?, page 17). Oils are composed of strings of short- and long-chain fatty acids. Palm oil, for example, contains five main fatty acids while coconut oil has eleven, and olive oil has six.

Those fatty acids have different properties that dictate the amount of lye necessary to turn the oil into soap. For example, palm oil is made of over 40 percent palmitic acid, a saturated fatty acid that makes palm oil solid at room temperature. Olive oil, however, contains up to 83 percent oleic acid, which is liquid at room temperature. Palm oil acts radically different than olive oil when mixed with sodium hydroxide, and the two oils require different amounts of lye to turn them into soap.

Fatty acids are also what give the final soap its different characteristics. For example, coconut oil promotes lather, while avocado oil is typically used to add nourishing characteristics to soap. Meadowfoam oil and mango butter both contribute conditioning and moisturizing properties, but the fatty acids in meadowfoam oil produce creamy bubbles while mango butter does not provide much lather.

The recipes in this book have all been carefully formulated to ensure a properly balanced bar of soap. If you are just starting out, it is best to follow all of the recipes exactly to get a feel for the process and what a good bar feels like. See chapter 7 to learn more about formulating your own recipes.

Balancing Oil and Lye

Soap works by laying down a slick of soapy lather that attaches to dirt. Both the lather and the dirt are rinsed away by water, but this process can also strip the skin of its natural oils and moisture. Extra oil in the soap can help to replenish the skin's natural oil barrier, making it feel moisturized.

This is why many soapers choose to leave a percentage of extra oil in their soap, a practice called "superfatting" or "lye discounting." A recipe that calls for the exact amount of lye necessary to convert all the oil into soap is said to have a zero percent lye discount or to be zero percent superfat. A bar that is zero percent superfat — meaning it has no excess oil after saponification — will be a stable, hard bar of soap, but it is likely to be somewhat less gentle to skin.

The downside of incorporating extra oils is that they can weigh down lather, decrease shelf life, and make a softer bar of soap that does not last as long in the shower. Superfatting is a personal preference. Most soapers choose to keep their superfat, or lye discount, to 10 percent or under. This book uses superfats between two and seven percent.

How Much Water to Use?

In addition to calculating the amount of each oil used in a given recipe, you also need to know how much water (or other liquid, depending on the recipe) is needed. The water acts as a carrier for the lye by forming ions that react with the oils. You need to use enough water to fully dissolve the lye, but not so much that it creates a sloppy bar of soap. Most calculators call for a range of water amounts, typically between 33 and 39 percent of the total amount of oil.

Using the maximum amount of water generally gives the best results. Using less water than the recipe calls for is called "water discounting." Soapers water-discount when they want to hasten the drying and curing time but still produce a hard bar of soap. If you use less water than the recipe calls for, your soap may reach trace (see page 14) more quickly than if the full water amount is used. If your soap becomes too thick too quickly, you will not have time to create elaborate designs. Water discounting is an advanced technique (see What Is a Water Discount?, page 63), best left until you have extensive experience soaping.

The Curing Process

Kevin Dunn, professor of chemistry and author of *Caveman Chemistry*, has determined that the bulk of the saponification reaction is finished in the first 24 hours. This does not mean, however, that you should use your soap within the first day.

Once soap has been unmolded and/or cut into bars, it must be set aside to cure and dry for four to six weeks in a well-ventilated area, turning bars every few days so that they dry evenly. This means if you make soap on January 1, your soap will not be ready to use, give away, or sell until January 29 at the earliest. During this period, the soap becomes more mild as the last traces of lye saponify and the bars lose weight as moisture evaporates, increasing hardness. This is important because a harder bar lasts longer in the shower.

Some Common Soapmaking Terminology

ACCELERATION. When the soap thickens quickly as the oils and lye-water are mixed. Often caused by components of fragrance and essential oils, it sometimes happens so fast the soap seizes up and is difficult to get out of the mixing bowl and into the container.

ALKALI. A strong base is required to saponify fixed oils. Sodium hydroxide (lye) dissolved in water is the alkali used to make bar soap. Potassium hydroxide makes liquid soap.

COLD-PROCESS. A soapmaking method that uses the heat created by the chemical reaction from mixing fixed oils, such as palm or olive, with lye.

CURE TIME/CURING. Most soaps should cure for four to six weeks after unmolding before being used. Curing allows water to evaporate, contributing to bar hardness and longevity, and often a milder final product.

FIXED OILS. Nonvolatile plant or animal oils comprising triglycerides and fatty acids. At room temperature they can be liquid or solid.

GEL PHASE. An optional phase in cold-process soapmaking where extra heat is produced to increase color vividness or bar hardness. Some fragrances and essential oils can cause gel phase without extra effort.

HOT-PROCESS. A method that, like cold-process, mixes oils and lye but also involves an external heat source. Hot-process soaping often utilizes crock pots or ovens as heat sources and the soap is fully neutralized once it has hardened. Liquid soap is also made this way.

LYE DISCOUNT OR SUPERFATTING. A reduction in the amount of lye called for in order to leave unsaponified oils in bar soap to provide extra moisturizing properties. The standard range of superfatting is between 2 and 10 percent.

SAP (SAPONIFICATION) VALUE. The amount of alkali needed to saponify a quantity of fixed oil. Each oil has a unique number, usually the average of a range.

SAPONIFICATION. The chemical reaction between triglycerides in fixed oils and an alkali solution. The alkali solution breaks the triglyceride into fatty acid salts — what we call soap — and glycerin.

SODA ASH. A white, powdery film of sodium carbonate that can form on soap when the lye and water react with carbon dioxide in the air, instead of the fixed oils in the soap. It is easily wiped off or rinsed away.

RICING. Caused by the addition of fragrance or essential oils that are not compatible with the soapmaking process. Sometimes accompanied by acceleration, ricing is different in that it creates small individual clumps of soap that look like rice granules. In cured soap, it can leave pock marks and oil pockets.

TRACE. The consistency of soap batter that signals emulsification of ingredients. It is identified by gently "tracing" a drizzle of batter on the surface; if the drizzle remains visible, the soap is said to be "at trace." Trace can range from thin (melted milkshake) to thick (pudding). Typically, colors and scents are added once trace is achieved.

WATER DISCOUNT. A reduction in the amount of water called for in a recipe in order to shorten the curing time and prevent soda ash. Typical water discounts are between 5 and 15 percent of the total. Reducing the water amount can accelerate the recipe.

The full cure time also helps to ensure that the lather of the bar is stable and long-lasting. Freshly made soap produces small, weak bubbles. Finally, if you are selling your soap, curing bars for the full time period is important to ensure that the final weight of the bar is correct and matches the label.

Soaping Safety Guidelines

It takes a powerful alkaline agent to turn oils into soap. For bar soap, this agent is sodium hydroxide, a common chemical that is found in any number of other applications, from cleaning drains to making face creams (even making pretzels, which are boiled in lye-water before baking!). Lye has an extremely high pH of 14.0. By comparison, lemon juice has a pH of around 2.0 and human skin has a pH of 5.0 to 6.0.

LYE IS CAUSTIC! It will burn skin, stain clothing, take the finish off wood, and damage many other surfaces. It can cause blindness and may be fatal if swallowed. Serious safety precautions must be taken when working with it, especially when it is dissolved in water.

A splash of lye-water will eventually eat through clothing and into your skin, leaving red marks and open sores. If you do spill lye-water on yourself, immediately remove contaminated clothing, including shoes, and wash your skin under cold running water for at least 15 minutes. (See Emergency Response on the next page.)

Many soapers keep vinegar on hand, believing it neutralizes lye burns. There is some controversy in the soapmaking community about washing lye burns with vinegar rather than water. Adding vinegar (an acid) to lye (a base) creates a chemical reaction that releases more heat. Additionally, the act of putting vinegar on a lye burn hurts. Just use water.

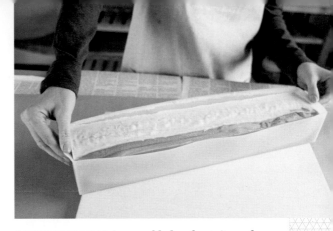

AFTER THE SOAP is unmolded and cut, it needs to cure for several weeks.

Although vinegar should not be used to treat lye burns on skin, it can be used as precaution during the cleanup process. A quick wipe of your workspace with a vinegar-soaked rag can neutralize any lye dust that may have gotten on the surface.

Working with Lye

When working with sodium hydroxide, **it is very important to follow these safety guidelines.**

1. *Always* use safety goggles that completely cover your eyes. **Glasses do not offer adequate protection — goggles are a necessity.** Some soapers wear a full-face shield.

2. Wear chemical-resistant gloves (see page 19 for more on protective wear). Best practice is to wear long sleeves, pants, and closed-toe shoes.

3. Mix the lye-water solution in a room with adequate ventilation. Add the lye slowly and carefully and stir gently. Do not breathe in the fumes. Some soapers use an air-filter mask.

4. Cover your workstation with cardboard or several layers of newspaper. Whenever possible, mix lye-water over a sink to contain spills and prevent accidents.

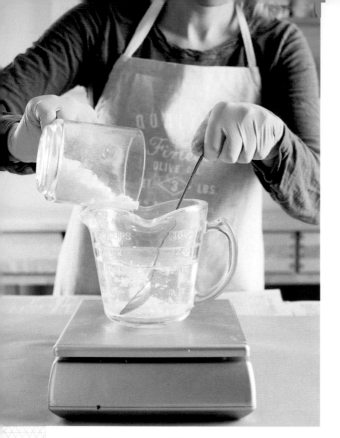

MIXING your lye solution

5. Mix your lye solution in a heat-safe container that is quite a bit larger than the amount of liquid you are mixing. When lye is mixed with water, it produces a heat reaction that goes up to 200°F (93°C). Other liquids (especially those containing sugars) can create an even warmer reaction.

6. **Always add the lye to the water, not the other way around.** Adding water to lye can create a caustic volcano that could foam out of the container.

Other Safety Precautions

Never soap with small children or pets in the room. Make sure they are adequately supervised so that you can give your full attention to your soapmaking process. It takes only seconds for a painful or debilitating accident to occur.

Avoid letting your soapmaking ingredients come into contact with aluminum, including containers, mixing utensils, and molds. It will ruin your soap and, worse, produce highly flammable hydrogen gas as a by-product.

Soap utensils are for soap. Food utensils are for food. Do not interchange soapmaking tools and food tools.

Emergency Response

SKIN. If you splash lye, lye-water, or fresh soap batter on any part of your body, immediately rinse the area with copious amounts of cold water. Then rinse some more, using fully cured soap to wash away the chemical residue. If you spill a large quantity on yourself, strip off your clothing at once and jump into a cold shower for 20 minutes, again using soap to clean off the lye. If your skin is red or painful after that, go to the emergency room.

EYES. Immediately flush with cold, running water for at least 20 minutes. Seek medical attention promptly.

THROAT. If you somehow swallow lye in any form, rinse your mouth thoroughly and then drink one or two large glasses of water. **Do not induce vomiting.** Seek immediate medical attention or call the American Association of Poison Control Centers at 800-222-1222.

What Is the SAP Value?

Saponification (SAP) values are expressed as the milligrams of potassium hydroxide (a slightly different version of lye used for liquid soapmaking) needed to saponify 1 gram of oil. Since exact fatty acid and triglyceride content of oils can vary from crop to crop, a range of SAP values is most often given. Since sodium hydroxide is used instead of potassium hydroxide to make bar soap, the original SAP value has to be converted for use in bar recipes.

Divide the potassium hydroxide SAP value of each oil in a given recipe by 1,402.5 to get the sodium hydroxide SAP value. Then add those SAP values to determine the total amount of lye needed.

The calculation looks like this:

POTASSIUM HYDROXIDE SAP VALUE ÷ 1,402.5 = SODIUM HYDROXIDE SAP VALUE

Typically either the average value in the SAP range or the lowest value is used; this example uses the low value. Here is a very simple soap that uses 1 ounce of each oil:

COCONUT OIL 250 ÷ 1,402.5 = 0.178

PALM OIL 202 ÷ 1,402.5 = 0.144

OLIVE OIL 188 ÷ 1,402.5 = 0.134

0.178 + 0.144 + 0.134 = 0.456 ounces of lye

Fortunately, you don't have to all this math by hand, as easy-to-use lye calculators are readily available online. See Using a Lye Calculator, to the right.

Using a Lye Calculator

The good news is that you never have to do soapmaking math by hand if you don't want to. There are a number of free lye calculators on the Internet that will calculate all your recipes with the click of a few buttons. Though they vary a bit in process, in general you enter the amounts of the oils you want to use, choose your preferred superfatting level, and click "Calculate" to get the correct amounts of water and lye needed for that recipe.

Some popular lye calculators are found at: www.brambleberry.com, www.the-sage.com, and www.summerbeemeadow.com. Many of these calculators allow you to resize recipes as well as formulate your recipes by percentages. There are also lye calculators available for smart phones.

Caution: Some lye calculators offer the option to create liquid soap recipes. Make sure that you are calculating for bar soap. Liquid soap uses a different form of lye (potassium hydroxide or KOH) and calls for different lye amounts. If you accidentally make bar soap using a liquid soap recipe, your soap will be lye heavy, making it extremely drying for skin or even dangerous to use.

CHAPTER 2

Choosing Equipment & Molds

*I*T TAKES ONLY a few basic tools to make a batch of soap. As you progress in your soapmaking journey, you can acquire additional tools that will make the process easier and allow you to create more elaborate designs. To start out, however, you need just a few things that can be found in a kitchen store or a thrift store.

When looking for equipment, think about long-term durability and safety. For example, wooden tools are not a good choice because they degrade over time and eventually can splinter in the soap. Choose heat-resistant glass bowls that are tempered to withstand repeated heating and exposure to lye.

Starting Out

The basic equipment for soapmaking can be found in any kitchen, but it's not a good idea to use your cookware to make soap. Buy a separate set of utensils and store them where they cannot be mistakenly used for food preparation.

You'll also need a large supply of newspaper or flattened cardboard to protect your entire work surface. If you don't have a dedicated soaping space, you can put a layer of heavy plastic under the papers to further protect your countertops.

PROTECTIVE WEAR. Lye-water and raw soap can burn and irritate skin and damage eyes. Protecting your eyes from start to finish is essential. Use goggles with a protective lip that fully covers your eyes (including your glasses, if you wear them) or use a full-face shield and air filter. This equipment can be found at a local hardware store. Wear gloves: the best type are disposable medical gloves (latex or nitrile), although you can use rubber dishwashing gloves. The tighter the fit, the less chance of clumsy mistakes.

A SCALE. Most ingredients in soapmaking, including liquids and oils, are measured by weight, not volume. Weight is more precise than volume, and in the science of soapmaking, precision matters. An inexpensive digital scale is easy and accurate, but a manual model works fine also. Choose a scale that can weigh heavy enough amounts for soaping. For example, don't get a scale that can't weigh amounts over 16 ounces if you plan on making large batches of soap.

MEASURING CUPS AND SPOONS. In addition to using them to measure ingredients, the cups are handy for coloring small portions of soap batter and for use as a design tool. A standard set of measuring cups works fine, but ones with pouring spouts are preferable. The longer the spout, the easier it is to do more elaborate designs. Measuring spoons are useful for ensuring precision with dry additives, such as exfoliants, colorants, and clays.

No Aluminum

THIS CAN'T BE STRESSED ENOUGH: Never use anything made of or containing aluminum to make soap. Aluminum reacts with sodium hydroxide to form hydrogen, a poisonous and explosive gas. At the very least, it will ruin your soap, and it could cause a serious accident.

Choose ones made of heat- and chemical-resistant material, never aluminum. Typically, fragrance and essential oils are weighed in glass containers. Some plastic containers can erode and degrade if used for pure essential or fragrance oils.

LYE-WATER CONTAINER. A heat-resistant measuring bowl (glass or plastic) with a handle and spout is critical for mixing water and lye and adding it to the oils. It's useful to have both a 2-quart and a 4-quart version; buy the larger one if you want to start with just one. It's important to allow plenty of headspace when mixing lye-water.

THERMOMETER. Monitoring the temperature of your ingredients is important. You want to be sure that delicate ingredients do not get scorched, to prevent soap volcanoes, and to ensure even emulsification and saponification. You can use a candy thermometer or a digital thermometer.

HEAT-RESISTANT BOWLS. You can use plastic, stainless steel, or glass bowls for mixing lye-water and soap batter, as long as they are heat- and chemical-resistant. Choose two or three bowls large enough to fit different-size soap batches with plenty of extra room — filling a bowl to the top, especially when mixing lye-water, invites spills that can burn you or ruin your countertops. Ideally, you should have 1-, 2-, and 3-quart capacity bowls on hand. Additionally, easy-pour containers with handles and long pouring spouts make it much easier to transfer the batter to the mold and perform delicate swirling techniques.

SPOONS, WHISKS, AND SPATULAS. You need at least one long-handled spoon for mixing batter and for creating designs. Whisks in a couple of different sizes are essential for mixing in fragrance oils and additives. They are also useful for maintaining the appropriate trace as you work. Spatulas are used to scrape the last of the soap batter out of mixing bowls and create intricate soap designs. Stainless steel is the ideal material for mixing utensils; silicone or heavy-duty rubber is acceptable. Over time, wood will degrade and splinter off into your soap.

STICK BLENDER. Also known as an immersion blender, this is a soapmaker's best friend. It reduces the tracing process from a 30- to 90-minute process to just a few minutes or even seconds, depending on your recipe. When choosing a stick blender, look for a model that will not whip much air into the soap. (I recommend those made by Cuisinart.) Buy one with a stainless steel shaft; a plastic shaft will eventually weaken and break. If the shaft detaches from the electrical unit, it is easier to clean.

Use Separate Soapmaking Tools

Technically, you could use equipment from your own kitchen to make soap, which, after all, is what is used to clean kitchenware, but it's worth repeating that this is not a good idea. Invest in a separate set of bowls, measuring cups, and other utensils and store them away from all equipment used for preparing food.

Unsaponified soap could get into crevices, and fragrances do leach into glass and plastic. Also, preparing food and soap using the same tools will not allow you to properly follow Good Manufacturing Practices set by the Food and Drug Administration (FDA).

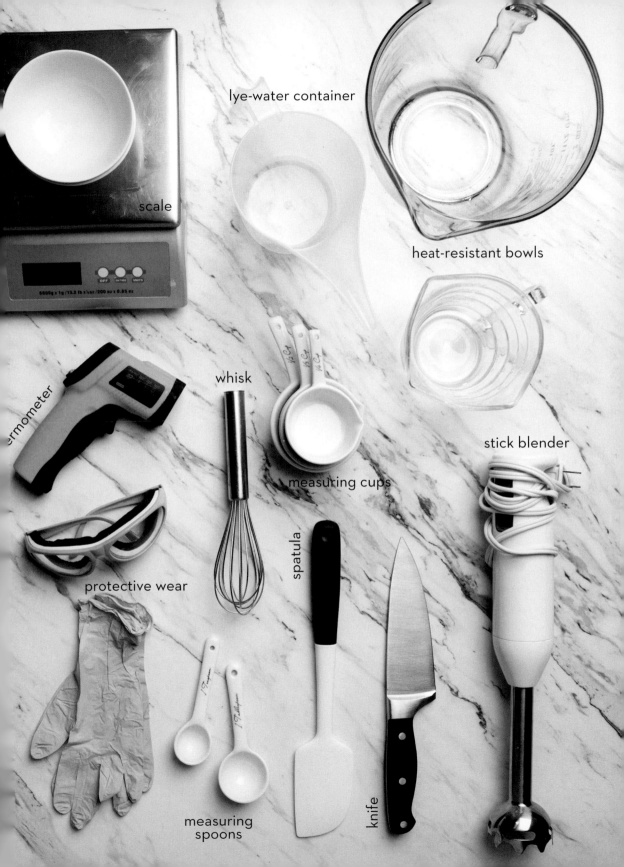

scale

lye-water container

heat-resistant bowls

thermometer

whisk

measuring cups

stick blender

spatula

protective wear

measuring
spoons

knife

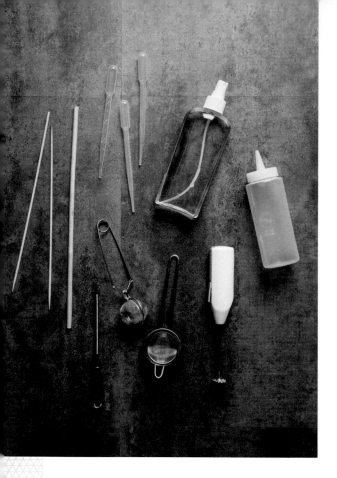

ISOPROPYL RUBBING ALCOHOL. Spraying 99% pure rubbing alcohol on your soap before it cures in the molds is optional, but it helps to prevent a layer of soda ash from forming on the surface of the bars.

SKEWERS OR CHOPSTICKS. These are used for making delicate swirls and designs in your soap. Wooden ones are fine in this case, as long as you wipe it off immediately after using to avoid degrading the wood. If cleaned quickly, skewers and chopsticks can last a long time.

FUNNEL. A funnel of any size is helpful for filling squirt bottles and is necessary for making complex designs such as the White Tea Faux Funnel Pour on page 118.

PLASTIC SQUIRT BOTTLES. Plastic condiment bottles are used for creating swirly, multilayered designs in soap. They help with accurate, even distribution of colors. You can also use them to store diluted lab colors. If you are using recycled containers, wash them thoroughly with soap and rinse with hot water before using for soapmaking.

EYEDROPPER OR SMALL PIPETTE. This is handy for precisely measuring fragrance and essential oils and for manipulating tiny amounts of soap batter to make designs.

DOUBLE BOILER. It is faster to infuse herbs and colorants using heat, and a double boiler allows you to evenly heat a larger amount of oil.

MINI MIXER. You can use the back of a spoon to mash powdered colorants into oil or water, but a mini mixer — often sold as a latte or milk frother — is handy for evenly and speedily mixing colorants and clays.

FINE-MESH STRAINER. A small strainer is useful for sprinkling pigments in layers to create designs.

KNIFE FOR CUTTING BARS. You can purchase a specially designed wire soap-cutter, but a sharp, non-serrated knife works just fine. A serrated knife will leave drag marks along the edges of your bars.

SMALL GLASS BOWLS. You can never have too many small glass bowls to hold measured amounts of additives, fragrance oils, essential oils, and colorants. Many ingredients, such as essential oils, are corrosive enough to damage plastic.

Other Useful Equipment

The following items aren't critical for making soap, but having them makes the process easier and more convenient. Some of these tools are necessary for making particular patterns or delicate designs.

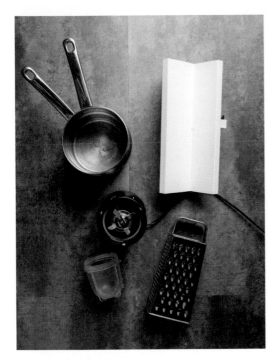

Selecting Different Molds

There are many options when thinking about molds for soapmaking. You can make your own from shoeboxes lined with freezer paper or reuse dairy-product containers and beverage cartons. You can utilize common kitchen containers (think Tupperware). Or you can buy wooden, plastic, or silicone molds made specifically for soap.

DIY Molds

As you get into soapmaking, you will start noticing many things around your house that appear to be fantastic options for soap molds. Yogurt and tofu containers, waxed-cardboard milk and juice cartons, the round tubes that potato chips and other snacks are sold in, and plastic food-storage containers (the kind that always seem to be missing their lids) — these all make excellent molds for soaps. Most of them can only be used once, though you can get more use out of sturdier plastic ones or by lining the molds with freezer paper.

Whatever you use needs to have some "give" to it, in order to release the soap after it has set. Metal and glass are not good materials for molds — the soap will stick and be nearly impossible to get out. Anything made of cardboard or wood must be lined with freezer paper. If you do want to use a particular metal mold, never use one made of aluminum, even if you are lining it.

Use only containers that held food or nontoxic materials. Before using a temporary soap mold, clean it thoroughly with soap and hot water.

Standard Molds

There are many sizes and shapes of soap molds on the market, and they come in a variety of materials. The two most common shapes are

SPICE/COFFEE GRINDER. A spice or coffee grinder is useful for pulverizing additives, including colors, to reduce clumping and make them easier to blend. A mortar and pestle also works.

MESH TEA BALL. A mesh tea ball is useful for straining unmixed clumps of colorants out of oils before soaping; for putting lines of colorant between layers; and for adding mica or herb toppings.

SOAP BEVELLER. This specialty tool creates clean 45-degree angles on your soap edges, giving them a professional appearance. You can use a vegetable peeler for close to the same effect.

CHEESE GRATER. A cheese grater is useful in shredding blocks of old soap to make rebatch soap or add confetti soap design elements.

vertical (tall and skinny) and horizontal (wide and flat). They create different bar shapes and offer different design options. Molds can be made of silicone, plastic, or wood. Raw wooden molds must be lined with either freezer paper or a silicone liner. Waxed paper will flake into your soap.

LOAF (OR LOG) MOLDS are typically used for impressive swirling, layering, and landscape designs. Loaf molds (wooden or silicone) come in all sizes, up to 95 pounds. When choosing a wooden mold, look for things that will help with unmolding, such as sides that flip down, or bottoms that slide out, or silicone inserts that fit in the mold. You can purchase specialty loaf molds made out of high-density plastic that do not require lining. They have their own set of challenges: they're often more expensive than wooden molds, soap can stick to the plastic, and depending on the material, they can expand and contract with heat. Many soap molds come with cutters that allow you to cut bars of even sizes.

A multi-pour sectioning tool is called for in some recipes that use this type of mold; it allows you to customize the look of your bars and create certain designs. It differs from standard dividers used in slab molds in that it is removed before the bars set up.

HORIZONTAL, SLAB, OR "DIVIDER MOLDS" provide a wider canvas for designs such as Lemon Linear Swirls (see page 90). Most horizontal molds come with optional dividers to form uniform bars that are easily unmolded. Horizontal molds are typically made from wood and need to be lined, though some are available in plastic. Dividers are typically made from a high density, heat-safe plastic.

SILICONE MOLDS — the kind commonly used for baking — are available in all shapes and sizes and work great for soap. They are less expensive than wooden molds, require no lining, and make unmolding easier, although it can be tricky to release soap as the soft sides make it possible to dent the bars. Choosing a recipe that is harder or using a soap-hardening agent such as salt or sodium lactate will help the unmolding process.

One downside is that silicone can produce pock marks in the final product if the soap overheats. To prevent this, keep your temperatures low (below 120°F [49°C]) when using silicone molds. Pock marks are solely aesthetic and do not affect the final feel or performance of the soap.

Specialty Molds

Specialty soap molds let you produce shapes you cannot achieve with other types of molds (say, a flying pig or a Celtic knot), so they are often worth the extra time and effort it takes to use them. Because they are made of heavy-duty plastic (HDPE or PVC), these molds have little flexibility, so unmolding them can be challenging.

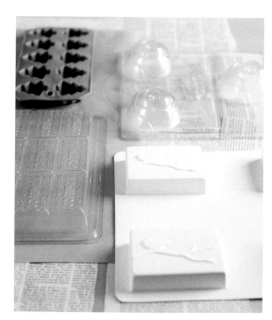

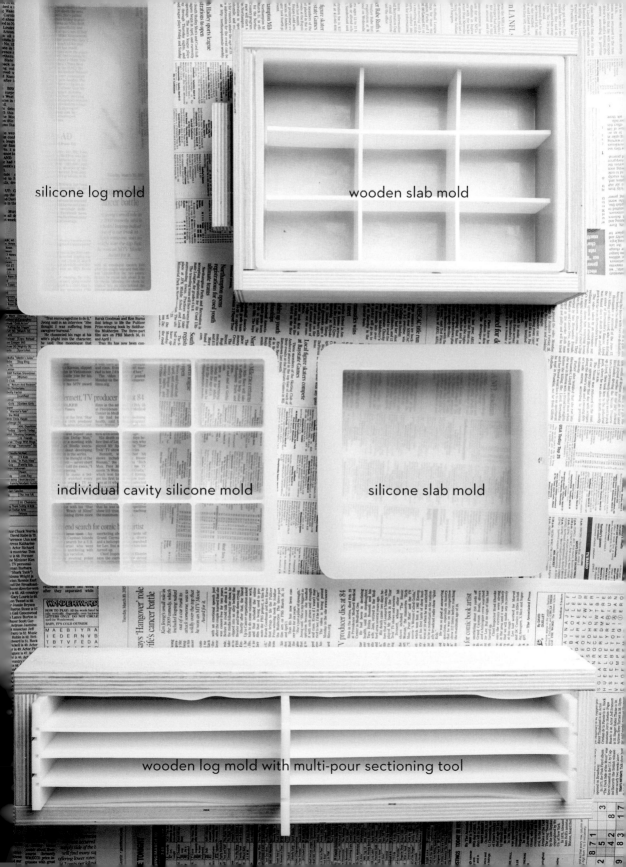

silicone log mold

wooden slab mold

individual cavity silicone mold

silicone slab mold

wooden log mold with multi-pour sectioning tool

They are best used with recipes for hard soap, or you can add sodium lactate to your lye-water to make the final bars easier to unmold. Another option is to lubricate the inside of the mold liberally with cyclomethicone (a liquid silicone) or a non-saponifying oil such as mineral oil. Cotton swabs can be handy for this process.

Candy molds or craft store quality molds that are made of thinner, less sturdy plastic can easily break during the soapmaking process. You can use them but if you do, choose a recipe that is extremely hard and be prepared to let the soap sit in the mold for a few extra days.

Some soap molds are designed specifically for creating embeds to put into larger batches of soap for interesting texture and patterns. Embeds need to be made ahead of the main batch, so those recipes take extra planning and time.

The Cleanup Process

Cleaning up after making soap is like cleaning any very oily pot or pan. It takes hot water and strong detergent, plus some elbow grease. Wear gloves while cleaning. **Remember:** The soap is still caustic and can burn you. Do not put soapy or oily soapmaking dishes in the dishwasher.

While it's tempting to use handmade soap for washing oily equipment, it takes a commercial detergent to cut down on major oil slicks in your plumbing. (Dawn is my favorite brand for this. There's a reason rescuers use it to clean off birds and other animals after oil-spill disasters.) Isopropyl rubbing alcohol is handy to have around — it cuts through grease when cleaning spills and wiping out soapmaking containers. Distilled vinegar can also be used to break up oil and wipe down the work surface once you are finished soaping.

1. Use a spatula to scrape any remaining batter out of the bowl into a soap mold. Wearing gloves, wipe leftover raw soap from bowls and utensils with paper towels; dispose of the towels in the garbage. Eliminating soap batter before washing utensils in the sink reduces the amount of oil and lye going down your pipes. Wiping up extra soap batter is especially important if your pipes are old, or you have a septic tank. While it is uncommon for soap batter oils to accumulate on pipes, it is possible.

2. Once excess soap has been removed, pile all containers, bowls, and utensils in an empty sink. Fill the sink with very hot water and a strong, grease-cutting detergent and let everything soak for a while. Start by washing the utensils with more detergent and a sponge reserved for soapmaking equipment.

3. To clean the stick blender, submerge the blades into a bowl filled with hot soapy water, and turn it on low speed for a few minutes to remove the soap inside the blender head. Rinse thoroughly with clean hot water. **Caution:** Never touch the blades of the stick blender to clean it without unplugging it.

4. Scrub the bowls and containers. Rinse thoroughly to ensure all soap is removed. Once finished, scrub the sink completely with commerical detergent and rinse with plenty of hot water.

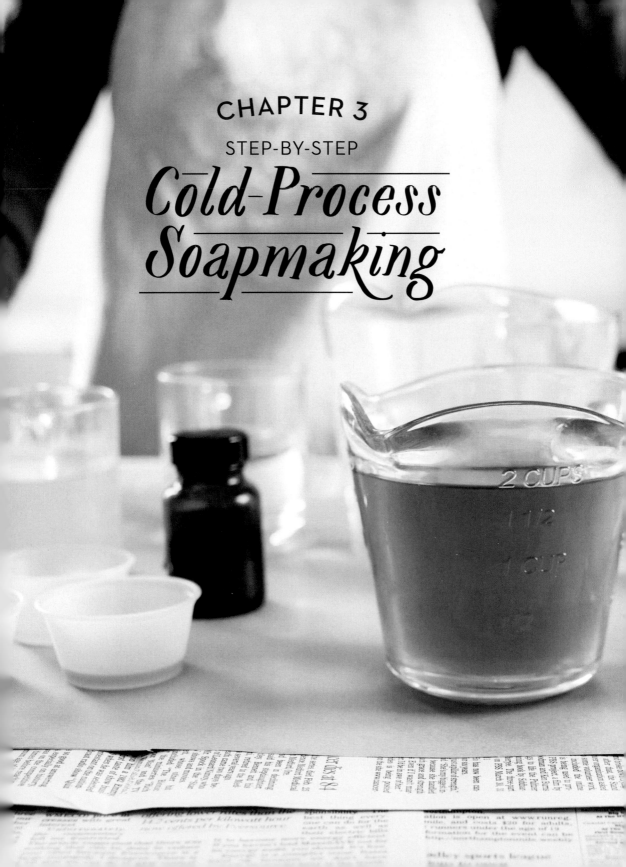

CHAPTER 3

STEP-BY-STEP
Cold-Process
Soapmaking

*I*F YOU HAVE NEVER MADE cold-process soap before, this is the perfect basic recipe to start with. It contains the three common soapmaking oils, and will make two pounds of soap or about eight beautiful, hard bars, depending on the type of molds you use. You can repurpose clean, dry plastic containers such as tofu or yogurt tubs — gather enough of them to hold 32 ounces of soap batter. If you use a larger container, you'll cut the final block into bars.

Before you begin, read the preceding chapters, collect your equipment, and set up a safe workstation. For a list of standard soaping equipment, see pages 19–22.

Lye-Water Amounts

3.0 ounces lye
(sodium hydroxide)

7.2 ounces distilled water

2 teaspoons sodium lactate
(optional)

Oil Amounts

5 ounces palm oil (23%)

5 ounces coconut oil (23%)

12 ounces olive oil pure
(54%) (See page 39.)

Colorant Amount

1/2 teaspoon yellow oxide
dispersed into 1/2 table-
spoon olive oil pure

Essential Oil Amount

1 ounce lemongrass
essential oil

Using Sodium Lactate

Most of the recipes in this book call for sodium lactate as an optional additive. Sodium lactate is a liquid salt that is naturally derived from the fermentation of sugars found in corn and beets. If you do not use it, your soap will turn out just fine, but adding it to cold-process recipes greatly reduces the time needed to unmold the soap.

The general usage rate is 1 teaspoon of sodium lactate for every 16 ounces (1 pound) of oils or 0.5 percent. It is stirred into the lye-water solution.

1. Measure the Lye-Water

Wearing gloves and goggles and working in a well-ventilated environment, weigh out the water in a heatproof container. Weigh out the lye flakes in a separate chemical-resistant container. Digital scales have a tare button, which tells the scale not to include a weight it is already measuring, such as the empty bowl. The easiest way to measure out ingredients is to use the tare button. To weigh multiple ingredients in the same container, use the tare button after the empty container is placed on the scale and again after each ingredient is added.

Slowly pour the lye into the water (never the reverse — the lye might bubble up like a volcano). Stir the mixture gently until the lye dissolves. If you are using sodium lactate, add it and stir to dissolve. Set the lye-water aside in a safe, out-of-the-way place to cool. It is ready to use when it has gone from cloudy to clear.

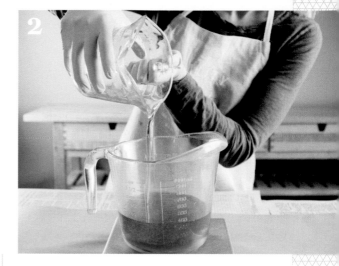

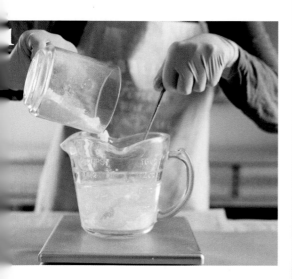

USE A CONTAINER that is somewhat larger than the total volume of lye-water called for.

2. Measure and Combine the Oils

Melt the palm oil in its original container, mix it thoroughly, and measure it into a bowl large enough to hold both the lye-water and the oils, with plenty of room left for mixing. (At room temperature, palm oil separates into fatty acids and other components, so it must be mixed separately every time to ensure equal distribution and a consistent product.)

Melt the coconut oil — either in the original package or by melting a glob of it in a separate bowl — then measure it, and add it to the soapmaking bowl. Add the olive oil and stir.

3. Mix the Soap

Check the temperature of the oils and lye-water. Unless otherwise noted, both temperatures should be under 140°F (60°C). Many soapers find a temperature range that feels the most comfortable for them and will work for most recipes. My personal preference is around 120°F (49°C), but every soapmaker has a different opinion.

Quick Melting Tips

When soaping with palm oil, it's important that the oil is thoroughly mixed in the container to incorporate all of the constituents before being added to soap. The quickest and most efficient way to do this is to melt those oils in their original container, then stir well before weighing out the amount needed. If the container is microwave-safe, heat the whole thing in short bursts at low power.

If you don't have a microwave, you can place the container of oil in a double boiler or hot-water bath (not over direct heat). This can be time consuming, as the water may need to be reheated to melt down the oil. Another option is to thoroughly stir together all of the solid and liquid elements of the palm oil in the container before weighing out the desired amount to melt.

Slowly add the lye-water to the oils, pouring it over the shaft of the stick blender or over a spatula to avoid adding bubbles to the mixture. You will be able to see a clear separation between the oils and the lye-water. Never pour the oil into the lye-water — it could cause a reaction that can bubble or splash over the sides of the container.

Achieving Trace

Place the stick blender on the bottom of the bowl. Tilt the bell of the blender sideways while fully immersed, and tap it on the bottom of the bowl to release any air bubbles. **Do not turn on the stick blender until it is fully submerged.**

Keep the stick blender on the bottom of the bowl and pulse it at high speed, mixing the oils and lye-water until they have reached thin trace, about 30 seconds.

NOTE: Each recipe in this book lists the specific time that it took to achieve the needed trace during testing. For most recipes, thin trace is achieved within about 30 seconds of stick-blending. Many factors contribute to trace times, including the starting temperatures of the ingredients, the power of your stick blender, and whether you blend straight through or pulse the stick blender. With all of these variables, it is important to learn to recognize the signs of trace. (See A Few FAQs, page 34.)

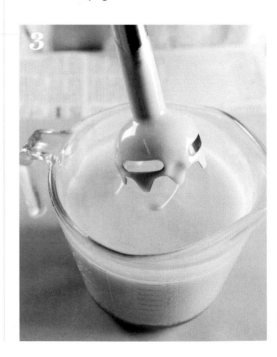

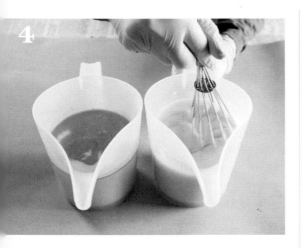

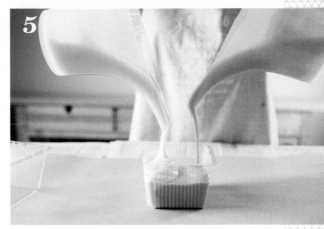

4. Mix in the Additives

Split the batter into batches, depending on the recipe directions. Add the essential oil and 1 teaspoon of the premixed colorant, and stir to combine. Many recipes call for using a whisk for this step, as using the stick blender at this point might accelerate trace too much.

5. Pour into the Mold

Prepare the mold as necessary. For this recipe, a simple container is divided into two sections, one for each color.

Pour the batter into the mold, scraping the edges of the bowl to make sure no soap is wasted.

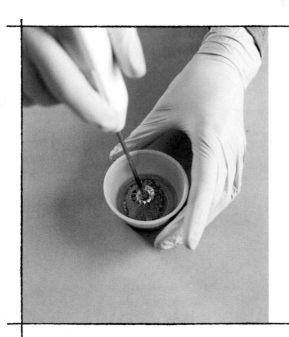

Preparing Colorants

Colorants typically come as powders that need to be mixed with oil in order to combine properly with the batter. Before adding a colorant, combine it thoroughly with a lightweight oil (amounts for both are given in every recipe), either whisking it by hand or using a mini mixer. The latter does a better job, but be sure to stir the powder into the oil a bit before turning on the mixer to avoid sending up a cloud of colored dust.

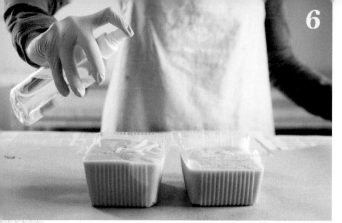

6. Mist with Alcohol

Lightly mist the top of the soap with 99% rubbing alcohol. The alcohol creates a barrier between the surface of the soap and the air, which helps to prevent soda ash.

Soda ash is a harmless by-product of soap that appears as a white, powdery substance across the surface. It is a purely an aesthetic flaw, and will not hurt the soap, so this step is optional.

7. Cover Mold

Place a folded piece of cardboard or similar item over the top of the mold so it isn't touching the soap, and cover the whole thing with a towel to insulate the soap. This technique is used in many soaps in this book to encourage gel phase. A soap that has gone through gel phase tends to have bolder colors and will harden more quickly. Not all soaps should go through gel phase, though. Soaps that contain additives with sugars, such as milks

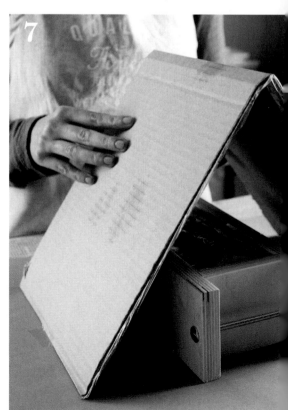

What Is Gel Phase?

Gel phase is the stage when a freshly poured soap heats up and begins to saponify as the lye reacts with the other ingredients. Soap typically gels when it reaches a temperature above 140°F (60°C) in the mold. Gelling begins in the center of the soap, where the heat is the most concentrated. The area that is in gel phase becomes dark, gelatinous, and somewhat translucent. As the soap cools, it begins to harden again and the colors become lighter and brighter. To gel or not to gel is personal preference which can vary from soap to soap.

Gel phase is a normal part of soap making. It happens naturally with most recipes that are mixed at 120°F (49°C) or above. It can also be created by higher initial starting temperatures of the lye-water and oils, additives (such as natural sugars) reacting with the lye, certain fragrance oils, and by placing the soap on a heating pad or insulating it to avoid heat loss.

Some soaps are enhanced by gel phase. Many of the natural colors in this book can only be achieved by fully gelling the soap, though there are some instances where gelling is not the best choice for a recipe. For example, most recipes containing milk are not gelled to avoid overheating and discoloring the milk.

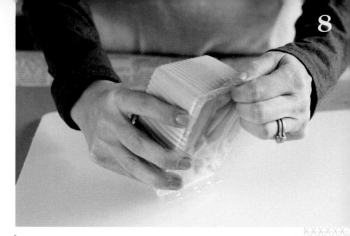

and purees, are naturally prone to heat up as the sugars react with the lye. These soaps are generally not insulated to avoid overheating the soap.

8. Unmold

Leave the soap in the mold for at least 48 hours before attempting to unmold it. Recipes differ in how long they take to set up. Formulas with a lot of soft oils (such as almond oil and olive oil) take longer than ones with a lot of hard oils (such as coconut, palm, or cocoa butter).

To unmold, gently pull the edges of the mold away from the soap to allow a little air in around the sides.

If the soap is not releasing smoothly or begins to tear or crack, do not force it. Allow the soap to set for another 48 hours and try again. (For tips, see Unmolding Stubborn Soap at right.)

9. Cut and Cure

Once the soap is unmolded, it can be cut into bars. The bar size and shape will depend on the container you used. Cut them so they fit comfortably in the palm of your hand. A sharp, nonserrated knife works well. Cut straight through the soap, and *slide* the soap off the knife, instead of pulling it off. This will prevent tearing the soap. If the soap is sticking badly to the knife or dragging, let it set for another few days on a well-ventilated rack (such as a cookie cooling rack) and try again after it has dried out some.

Let the soap cure in a well-ventilated area for 4 to 6 weeks before using or selling the bars. Turn the bars every few days to ensure they cure evenly. During the cure time, excess moisture will evaporate, the bars will become more mild to use and the lather will improve.

Unmolding Stubborn Soap

All of the recipes in this book include sodium lactate as an optional ingredient, because it can greatly speed up the time needed for a soap to unmold easily. If you choose to leave it out, your soap may take a bit longer to unmold. There are other reasons why a soap may be difficult to unmold — one of the most common is the type of oils used. Over half of the recipes in this book contain no palm oil, which is a hard oil that helps soap set up faster. If the recipe uses other oils and is difficult to unmold, wait a few days and try again.

If you just cannot wait to get your soap out of the mold, you can pop any soap that is at least 24 hours old into the freezer overnight so the soaps retract a bit from the sides of the mold. For the best unmolding success, hold the mold on one corner with both hands and gently pry the mold away from the side of the soap. Do this for all four corners, or until the soap breaks free and can be slid out. Some soap stays stuck in the mold for weeks. Be patient if this happens — you don't want to break your mold to release the soap.

A Few FAQs

Why do I need to use distilled water?

Distilled water makes longer-lasting bars of soap. Tap water often contains additives such as chlorine, minerals, and even heavy metals from the piping system. Minerals and heavy metals can cause DOS (Dreaded Orange Spots) in your soap. While DOS is safe, it can ruin a beautiful batch of soap with its unattractive appearance and off-putting odor.

Lye is so caustic; why is it necessary?

Soap is a combination of oils or fats, and lye. Without the latter, the oils will not go through the chemical reaction required to produce soap. In a properly calculated recipe, the lye reacts completely with the oils, leaving none in the final bar of soap. All of the recipes in this book produce final bars that have no trace of residual lye. Soaps that are advertised as "lye free" are likely not true soaps and are usually labeled as "beauty bars," "cleansing bars," or something similar. These products are typically created from surfactants, chemicals that act as degreasers.

What exactly is "trace"?

The word "trace" comes from the idea of literally tracing a design — or your name, even! — into the soap batter after mixing it. To determine the degree of trace, drizzle a line of batter off your stick blender over the pot of soap.

THIN TRACE appears when the oils and lye-water are completely combined with no visible oil streaks or pockets and the batter is just beginning to thicken, similar to a melted milkshake texture. When batter at thin trace is drizzled on the surface of the mixture, the drizzle does not immediately sink, but remains visible for a few seconds.

MEDIUM TRACE is when the batter moves from melted milkshake texture to more of a cake batter texture. This is the ideal stage for mixing in additives, such as poppy seeds, that need to remain suspended in the batter, and to create layers of soap that need to support additional layers. You should be able to "trace" a few letters on the surface before the first letter sinks into the batter.

THICK TRACE is when the batter develops into a thick pudding texture, and holds its shape when spooned or poured out. Thick trace is great for creating textured tops and holding up embeds.

NOTE: It is better to stop blending and check if you aren't sure how thick your trace is; you can always thicken it, but you cannot make it thinner!

What might prevent soap from achieving trace?

One factor is that not all stick blenders are equal. The recipes in this book use the amount of time that it took to achieve trace with Cuisinart brand stick blender. If your stick blender has less power, it will take longer than the suggested trace time. Blend for a little longer to see if it starts to pull together.

If your stick blender is not the problem, then run through your ingredient list to ensure that you used the proper amounts of oils, lye, and liquid. The most likely reasons that soap will not trace are too much oil too much water or not enough lye. If the proper amounts of pure ingredients are used, your batter will turn into soap every time. Stick-blend for longer, up to five minutes.

Hot-Process Hero to the Rescue

Sometimes a batch of soap just refuses to trace. Common reasons for this are mixing by hand instead of using a stick blender; using lye that isn't fresh or using potassium hydroxide instead of sodium hydroxide; or making mistakes when measuring ingredients. It is possible to save a problem batch, but it's tricky. Set aside a couple of hours, put on your safety gear, and give this a try:

1. Pour the separated batter into a stainless steel pot large enough so that the soap only fills it about one-third full.

2. Put the pot on the stove on medium-low and stir the gloppy mess frequently until it turns more solid — about the consistency of mashed potatoes. This can take 15 minutes to 1 hour. Do not leave the pot unattended.

3. Glop the soap into molds and wait at least 48 hours or until it is hard enough to unmold. Dry the bars for the usual 4 to 6 weeks.

Dumping a Bad Batch

If you can't salvage your soap, scrap it into a disposable container and let it cool and harden as much as possible before triple bagging it in plastic bags and disposing of it in the trash.

If you still have not achieved trace, there is a chance that you will not. However, go ahead and pour it into the mold and see if it hardens. If the problem is too much water, it will eventually evaporate.

What is the white, powdery stuff on my finished soap?

Soda ash is a very common, harmless substance that forms on cold-process soap when a small amount of unreacted lye in newly poured soap reacts with carbon dioxide. It can easily be prevented by spraying the mold with 99% rubbing alcohol to create a barrier while the soap sets up.

A number of factors can contribute to soda ash: two common ones are the temperature of the soap (cold soap tends to ash more than gelled soap) and trace that is too thin. To prevent ash, keep the temperature of the soap at 120°F (49°C) or more (unless otherwise specified for a recipe) and make sure your soap is at a full trace where you can easily see trailings on the surface of the batter.

Another factor is too much water in the batter, so experienced soapers may choose to remove 10 percent of the recommended liquid from a recipe for an effective fix. Note that using a water discount causes the soap to have less working time. Some soapers also add a very small amount of melted beeswax at high temperatures (above 140°F [60°C]) at thin trace to lessen soda ash.

CHAPTER 4

All about Oils

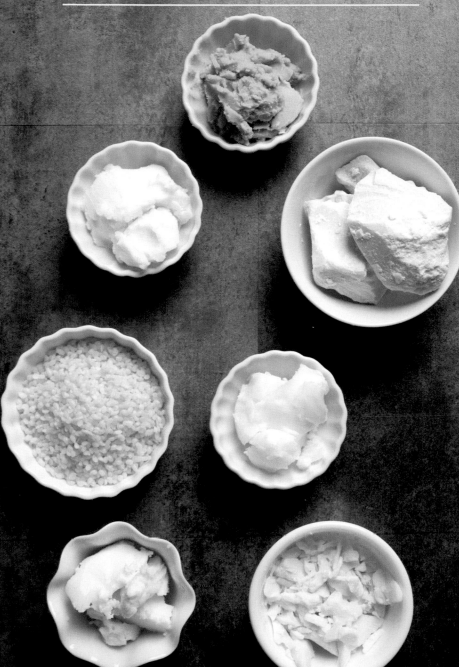

MANY DIFFERENT OILS can be used to make soap. Each one imparts different qualities to the final product. For example, an oil that is high in saturated fats has good lathering properties and adds to bar hardness; an oil that is high in unsaturated fats helps with moisture and conditioning. This chapter describes a number of oils that are commonly used in soapmaking.

Apricot Kernel Oil

(SAP VALUE: .135)

Apricot kernel oil comes from the kernels (seeds) of the fruit. It is high in fatty acids and vitamins A, C, and E. It is also high in unsaturated fat, which means that it adds to conditioning and moisturizing properties, but does not help with cleansing or bar hardness. Apricot kernel oil is typically used at 15 percent or less in soapmaking recipes.

Avocado Oil

(SAP VALUE: .133)

Avocado oil is a heavier oil pressed from the pit of the avocado. Depending on the type of extraction, the color varies from green to yellow, which has little effect on the color of the final product. Avocado oil adds to conditioning and moisturizing properties in soap. It is typically used at 20 percent or below in recipes.

Canola Oil

(SAP VALUE: .133)

Canola oil is an economical soaping oil that is fantastic when a recipe needs a lot of working time or a neutral color. High oleic canola oil is the best choice as it will not go rancid as quickly as traditional canola oil. Canola oil is best used in conjunction with hard oils such as coconut and palm oil. It can be used up to 40 percent in soapmaking recipes.

Castor Oil

(SAP VALUE: .128)

Castor oil, an extract of the castor bean plant, is a thick, sticky oil with a distinctive odor. It is light yellow in color, but this doesn't typically affect the color of the final product. Castor oil creates large, luxurious bubbles, but is typically used at 8 percent or below in recipes to avoid tackiness.

Cocoa Butter

(SAP VALUE: .137)

Cocoa butter is extracted from the cacao bean. It has a distinctively nutty, chocolate-y aroma and is used in making chocolate. Despite its name, it has a hard and crumbly consistency and must be melted before being mixed with lye-water. Cocoa butter comes in two forms, deodorized and natural. The deodorized version, sometimes called Maria grade, is usually whiter than natural cocoa butter and does not smell like chocolate.

When used in cold-process soap, cocoa butter contributes to bar hardness. If it's used over 15 percent, the soap may become difficult to cut and be prone to cracking. The soap may also take on a slight cocoa fragrance.

Coconut Oil

(SAP VALUE: .178)

Used in cooking, baking, and soapmaking, coconut oil is typically expeller pressed from the meat of coconuts, then bleached and deodorized. Coconut oil extracted with solvents is less desirable. Coconut oil has a variety of melt points: 76°F (24°C), 96°F (35.5°C), 101°F (38°C), and 110°F (43°C). They all work for soap, but the 76°F–melt point version is the most commonly used.

Coconut oil creates lather with large bubbles and helps to cut down on oils and grease. It has a high cleansing ability, so some find it harsh on the skin if used above 25 percent. Its long shelf life and high stability make it a staple in soapmaking.

Coffee Butter
(SAP VALUE: .132)

Coffee butter is a luxurious butter that smells just like a slightly burnt cup of coffee. It is a blend of coffee seed oil and hydrogenated vegetable oils, giving it a soft, buttery application. Pale brown in color, it can impart a lovely natural tan color into the final soap, as well as a subtle roasted coffee scent. Coffee butter contains between 0.5 and 1 percent natural caffeine. It has a shelf life of about one year. It does not contribute much to the lather or hardness of the bar, but is considered moisturizing. It is typically used at 10 percent or less.

Hempseed Oil
(SAP VALUE: .135)

Hempseed, or just hemp, oil, does not contain tetrahydrocannabinol (THC), a psychoactive constituent found in the seeds. Depending on the degree of refining, its color varies from light yellow to dark green. It is used in skincare products because of its high proportion of essential fatty acids.

In soap, it provides a nourishing yet small lather. Shelf life can vary depending on the type of refining. Unrefined hempseed oil has a short shelf life of 3 to 6 months. Refined hempseed oil has a shelf life of 12 months. It is typically used at 20 percent or less in soapmaking recipes.

Macadamia Nut Oil
(SAP VALUE: .194)

Macadamia nut oil has a rich feeling on skin and may be used in heavy moisturizing creams. In soap and cosmetics, it is often used to replace mink oil, which many people prefer to avoid. It is stable in soapmaking, although it does not produce copious bubbles. Macadamia nut oil provides conditioning and moisturizing qualities. Because it does not contribute much to bar hardness or lather, it is typically used at 10 percent or less.

Mango Butter
(SAP VALUE: .137)

Mango butter comes from the seed of the mango fruit. The seed is pressed, and the resulting oil is refined, bleached, and deodorized until it is ivory in color with a creamy texture. It has a shelf life of 6 months to a year. In soap, it adds conditioning and nourishing properties. It is typically used at 15 percent or less in soap recipes.

Meadowfoam Oil
(SAP VALUE: .120)

Meadowfoam oil is derived from the seeds of the meadowfoam plant (*Limnanthes alba*). It is unusual in having almost 100 percent long-chain fatty acids, which makes it extremely emollient and moisturizing. Meadowfoam has a shelf life of up to three years when stored in a refrigerator. Because it does not add to bar hardness or lather, it is typically used at 20 percent or less. Using more produces a slightly softer bar with smaller bubbles.

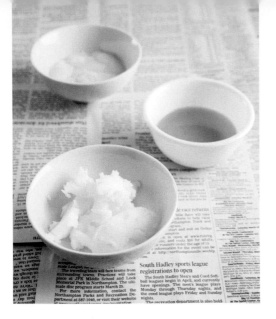

Olive Oil

(SAP VALUE: .134)

Olive oil is available in a variety of grades. While extra-virgin olive oil is not necessary for soap recipes, it is important to use a pure grade. Some methods of extraction, such as the last pressing, include the use of chemical solvents, which may be present in the final product. These chemical solvents can lead to acceleration of trace.

EXTRA-VIRGIN OLIVE OIL (OLIVE OIL PURE) allows for a very long working time, and is a staple for designs with complicated swirls, lots of different colors, or accelerating essential oils, such as cinnamon. If a recipe calls for olive oil pure, it is best not to substitute with olive oil pomace, which will trace more quickly.

OLIVE OIL POMACE is made by removing the last bits of oils and fats from the paste left over from pressing extra-virgin olive oil. It contains high percentages of unsaponifiables, and is known to speed up trace. This oil is used when a recipe needs to set up slightly sooner, such as in some of the layering projects, or recipes that have

a textured top. Extra-virgin olive oil can be substituted in these recipes, but be aware that the trace times will be longer.

All types of olive oil produce an exceptionally mild soap with small bubbles, suitable for sensitive skin and babies. Unlike other oils, it can be used up to 100 percent in soap recipes. When fresh, the lather is slick. Olive oil soap ages beautifully, improving its lather over time.

CAUTION: The exception is "light" olive oil, which often doesn't work in soap at all.

Palm Oil

(SAP VALUE: .144)

Palm oil comes from the pulp of the fruit from palm trees. In soap, palm oil helps to stabilize lather, adds to making a harder bar of soap, and acts as a secondary lathering agent. When used in conjunction with coconut oil, the lather is stable and large. Because of its hardening ability, palm oil should be kept to 25 percent or less of your recipe. For soapmaking, look for RBD (refined, bleached, deodorized) palm oil.

Palm oil is becoming increasingly controversial because of its environmental impact (see What Is Sustainable Palm Oil?, on the next page). Over half of the recipes in this book don't use it, so although palm oil is a wonderful oil for soap, it is not required.

Palm Kernel Oil

(SAP VALUE: .178)

Palm kernel oil (PKO) is obtained from the kernel (the nut-like core) of the palm plant. PKO comes as flakes and is solid at room temperature. It contains highly saturated fats that contribute to bar hardness in soap and lather stability. When used at amounts higher than 15 percent in soap, it will accelerate trace and the soap can become brittle and waxy.

What Is Sustainable Palm Oil?

Palm oil is grown in a number of South Asian and African countries. The plantations require massive amounts of land to keep up with the demand, and some unscrupulous plantations illegally clear surrounding rainforest and peat, leading to the destruction of orangutan and other wildlife habitat. Certified Sustainable Palm Oil (CSPO) is sourced from plantations that do not log in primary forests or areas of biodiversity or endangered species.

The Roundtable on Sustainable Palm Oil (RSPO) oversees CSPO certifications. In addition to ensuring that habitat is not being destroyed, the organization works to reduce the use of pesticides and fires for clearing, and advocates for the fair treatment of workers according to the international labor rights standards. If you would like to use palm oil in your soap but are concerned about the harmful effects of unsustainable palm harvesting, ask your vendor if they source RSPO-certified palm oil.

Peach Kernel Oil

(SAP VALUE: .135)

Peach kernel oil is rich in vitamin E, making it a great addition for mature skin. A light oil, it is typically a pale, neutral color. Peach kernel oil contributes to a stable lather when used with coconut oil, but it does not add to bar hardness. Though it can be used up to 25 percent, it is typically used in smaller amounts.

Rice Bran Oil

(SAP VALUE: .129)

Rice bran oil is derived from the outer layers of rice: the bran and the germ. These layers are packed with antioxidants, essential fatty acids, and vitamin E. It produces small, mild lather, similar to olive oil, and can be used in place of olive oil to lower bar cost. Though it can be used in cold-process recipes up to 100 percent of the oils, it is typically used at 50 percent or below.

Safflower Oil

(SAP VALUE: .135)

Safflower oil is an inexpensive oil that is moisturizing in soap and creates a mild, low lather. It can be used interchangeably with sunflower or canola oil (after running through a lye calculator). Standard safflower oil has a fairly short shelf life of one year, so look for the high oleic version to increase the shelf life. It can be used up to 25 percent in recipes.

Shea Butter

(SAP VALUE: .128)

Shea butter is produced from the nut of the African shea tree. In its most unrefined state, it is a gray, smoky-smelling product. When fully refined, bleached, and deodorized, it turns creamy and white.

In soap, shea butter has great moisturizing abilities, and because it is a well-known ingredient, it provides ample label appeal. It is not a good lathering agent on its own, and can speed up trace. It is typically used at 10 percent or below in most soapmaking recipes.

Soybean Oil

(SAP VALUE: .135)

Soybean oil is available as a liquid and as a hydrogenated (solid) oil. Both add to the conditioning properties of soap. Because of its price, soybean oil is an attractive filler oil for soap recipes. It produces a mild and thin lather. Though it has a shelf life of up to 12 months, liquid soybean oil does not contribute to bar hardness. It is typically used at 50 percent or less in a recipe.

Sunflower Oil
(SAP VALUE: .134)

Sunflower oil is full of essential fatty acids and vitamin E, which condition and moisturize skin. It has a short shelf life, so either keep it in the fridge or look for high-oleic versions, which tend to be more stable. When combined with olive and palm oil, it helps to produce a rich, creamy lather. Use sunflower oil at less than 20 percent in soap recipes, or it will result in a soft soap.

Sweet Almond Oil
(SAP VALUE: .136)

Sweet almond oil is a food-grade oil pressed from edible almonds (*Prunus amygdalus* var. *dulcis*), not the poisonous bitter almond (*P. amygdalus* var. *amara*). Sweet almond oil has many vitamins, including A, E, and B$_6$. It contributes to conditioning and moisturizing skin, but will make softer bars. It is typically used at 25 percent or less and has a shelf life of 9 to 12 months.

Using Animal Fat Instead of Oil

Many soapers, especially those who raise livestock, prefer to soap with rendered animal fats in place of vegetable oils. Animal fats have been used for hundreds of years in soapmaking and they can create wonderful bars of soap that are very hard and white bars with mild, creamy lather. Tallow and lard, from beef and pork respectively, are the most common, although some soapers have been known to use more exotic fats, such as bear or beaver.

The fat from any type of animal may be used, although they will all have slightly different SAP values, generally within the range of .134 to .141. Tallow has a SAP value of .138 to .141; lard's is .139–.141. There are a few outliers, such as lanolin, with a SAP value of .075, and mink oil, with a SAP value of .160. Always check the exact SAP value for any fat, or use a lye calculator; small differences in SAP value can have a big effect on the amount of lye needed to turn the fat into soap.

Considering Nut Allergies

When making soap for other people, it's important to be aware of nut allergies. Depending on the severity of an individual's allergies, the use of nut-based oils (and other nut-derived ingredients such as exfoliant shells, described in chapter 5) can cause adverse reactions. Here are some of the more commonly used nut oils that might cause a problem for certain individuals. When labeling soap for sale, make sure to list every ingredient used in the soap — including carrier oils and oils used to disperse colorants — to help keep customers with allergies safe.

» Almond oil (sweet almond oil)

» Hazelnut oil

» Macadamia nut oil

» Peanut oil

» Walnut oil

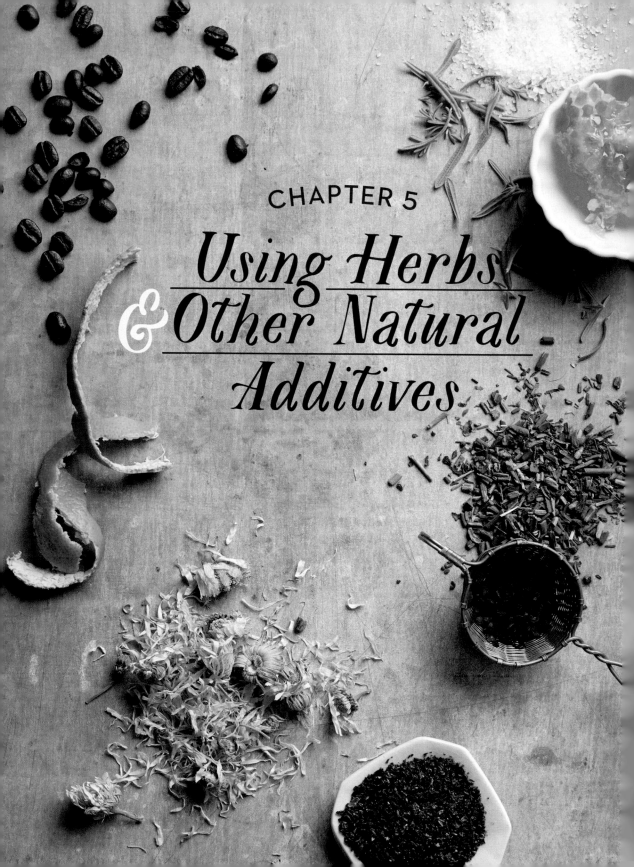

CHAPTER 5

Using Herbs & Other Natural Additives

T HE USE OF NATURAL INGREDIENTS in body care products, long a popular commercial trend, continues to increase. Adding herbs and other natural additives can increase customer demand, label appeal, and overall aesthetics. Additives such as herbs and flowers, coffee and tea, nuts, chocolate, oatmeal, silk fibers, and even tobacco can be added for many different reasons. For starters, many of them have excellent antioxidant properties, which can help to increase the skin-loving traits of your bar. Others make for great use as exfoliants. They can also help to color your soap or add texture.

Before You Start

When adding natural products to soap, there are a few things to take into consideration:

Will it discolor?
While some herbal additives produce beautifully colored soap, most others will eventually turn brown and discolor the final product. Some cause a "halo" effect where the color spreads out from the herb particles in the soap, eventually taking over most of the bar. You'll want to plan for this when creating your soap design. Or just use those soaps up more quickly!

How scratchy will it be?
If you're using additives as an exfoliant, you'll want to do some testing to find the correct "scratch factor." A product that is ground too finely or used in very small amounts will be unnoticeable; using larger chunks or adding too much of it could potentially cause harm. (Nobody wants to lose a layer of skin!)

Is this additive a possible allergen?
Additives like nutshells could cause an allergic reaction in some sensitive people. You'll want to make sure you add a warning to your label if using any of these. (See Considering Nut Allergies, page 41.)

Should I use the herb itself or make an infusion?
When using herbs to color your soap, you'll need to make an oil infusion to extract as much colorant as possible. To use them as an exfoliant, to add texture, or for aesthetic purposes, adding the actual herb directly at thin trace is fine. (See pages 48–49 for directions on making herbal infusions.)

How long will natural colors last in soap?
How long color lasts depends on the ingredient. Natural green colors tend to fade fairly quickly (within a couple of weeks) to brown or gray or even become almost non-existent. Shades of orange and red, such as the tomato color in Layered Tomato Swirl Bars (page 126) will fade, but not as drastically or as quickly as the greens.

Keeping your soap out of direct sunlight can help extend the life of the color. A good alternative to natural colorants is to use nature-identical oxides, which are often called for in this book. They hold their color much better.

USING HERBS & OTHER NATURAL ADDITIVES

A Word from the FDA

Depending on its labeling and intended use, a botanical product can be considered a food, a dietary supplement, a drug, and/or a cosmetic. While it is possible to incorporate nearly any botanical item into your product, the FDA has differing rules for how they can be used. Specifically, many herbs and additives can be used for their healing or supportive properties but are not approved for use as colorants, even though many herbs (and other additives, such as clay) impart lovely colors to soap.

For example, spirulina makes your soap turn green. However, the FDA has only approved spirulina as a colorant in the narrow category of candy, gum, and confection. If you just want green soap for personal use, you don't have to worry about this. But if you use spirulina in soap that you plan to sell, you must add it for the herbal properties and not its natural green color.

Do your research on the therapeutic properties and approved FDA uses of your chosen ingredients, so that you don't run up against labeling laws. Labeling your product with any claims such as "warming" or "healing" or "anti-aging" requires following the requirements of the FDA for production of a drug rather than a cosmetic.

Some Common Additives

There are dozens, if not hundreds, of herbal, mineral, botanical, and other materials that can be added to soap to create colors, impart specific characteristics, and increase the appeal of the final product. Here are just a few that are used in recipes in this book.

CLAYS are used to impart color to soap (see All About Color, page 46, and Using Clay to Color Soap, page 49) and can also add "drag" (mild exfoliating property) or "slip" (a slick feeling), depending on the type of clay used. This makes clay soap an excellent shaving bar but may surprise people who are using clay bars for the first time. Additionally, clay is a strong odor-masking agent. This makes it ideal for deodorizing soap but less ideal if you prefer to smell the essential oil in your soap.

COFFEE GROUNDS are a great additive for a super exfoliating bar. They can be ground to whatever texture you desire. For extra scrubbing power, use a coarse grind, while for gentle exfoliation, a super-fine espresso grind is best. Use the grounds to make coffee before adding them, or they might bleed brown halos into the final soap.

COLLOIDAL OATMEAL has long been used as a soothing bath additive. It is ground micro-fine, and is extremely gentle, giving just a hint of texture in the final bar without being scratchy. It usually appears slightly gray in the final soap. Adding colloidal oatmeal can accelerate trace in your soap recipe; premixing with water can help avoid this.

HONEY can be tricky as a soap additive, but it can create some wonderful results. Honey is known for its antimicrobial properties as well as its humectant abilities, and sugar in general enhances lather. While sugar can impart some fantastic properties to your soap, it also introduces factors to work around. Sugar and lye react to create excess heat, which can cause extreme gel phase, sweating, cracking, heat tunneling (large holes in the center of the soap), or even make the soap erupt from the mold. To work with honey, start soaping with lye-water and oils both under 100°F (38°C). Add the honey at trace, and stick-blend in short bursts to disperse it into the batter. Once the soap is finished, place it in the refrigerator or freezer immediately to prevent overheating.

OXIDES AND PIGMENTS are called for throughout this book to add color in recipes. These dry powders are much more easily incorporated into soap batter when mixed into a light oil such as sweet almond or rice bran oil. The standard ratio is 1 part oxide to 3 parts oil. You can mix the color and oil together with a spoon, but an electric mini mixer such as a latte frother is wonderful to ensure there are no chunks of color in the mixture. Store extra colorant in the refrigerator and discard after one month. (Read more about oxides and pigments on the next page.)

SALT is a versatile additive that creates an extremely hard and white bar. Sea salt is commonly used for soap as it contains many minerals and creates label interest. Salt decreases lather significantly, so a very cleansing, high-lathering oil such as coconut oil may be needed for balance. Salt can be added at trace to create an exfoliating textured bar, or to the lye-water (see 100% Castile-Brine Stamped Cube, page 74). Salt-added soap is best made in an individual cavity mold, as a loaf becomes too hard and brittle to cut without damaging the bars.

TUSSAH SILK is made of very fine, soft fibers harvested from wild silkworms. Adding silk to your soap creates a slick, soft feel to the lather, and many soapers will not soap without it. To use it, add a very small pinch of the fibers to the water before the lye is added. Pour the lye directly over the silk and stir continuously. The fibers will begin to dissolve as you stir. Once the silk is dissolved, continue with the recipe as usual. The fibers can be added to any recipe and will not affect the final appearance of the bar.

WALNUT SHELLS can be found pre-ground at many soap suppliers. They are typically finely ground for skin care, and make an excellent facial soap. They do not bleed color, but will appear as brown flecks in the final bar.

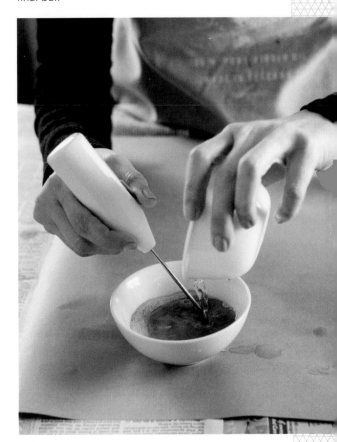

USING A MINI mixer ensures that clay and other additives are evenly mixed before being added to soap batter.

Using Herbal Extracts

Herbal extracts are a great way to add antioxidants and vitamins from plants into your soaps. Extracts for soaping are oil- or water-based liquids that contain the active ingredients of an herb in a concentrated form. Alcohol-based extracts, such as tinctures or baking extracts, can have adverse, possibly dangerous, reactions in the soaping process, so they should not be used. Some oil-based extracts are also effective colorants that give your soaps some pop without using synthetic alternatives.

Extracts are made by infusion or decoction. Making infusions and decoctions is easy; the methods differ only slightly. To make an infusion, submerge the herb, typically leaves and other soft plant matter, in very hot liquid and let it steep for a while (see Making Herbal Oil Infusions to Color Soap, page 48). Bark, seeds, and other dense, hard material must simmer for an extended period of time to extract their active ingredients; after straining out the material, the resulting liquid is a decoction.

Please note that these are not baking extracts, but botanical extracts specifically prepared for their herbal properties. Baking extracts are often alcohol-based and should never be used in soapmaking. Botanical extracts may be added to cold-process soap to enhance or increase the therapeutic properties, for antioxidant properties, or to add label value.

Add the extract at thin trace for the best chance of the extract making it through the saponification process. There is some debate in the soapmaking community as to whether the constituents in extracts survive. Because of this, many soapers prefer to use extracts in hot-process or rebatch soap where the delicate extract is not exposed to active lye. When the main purpose of using an extract is to add color (see Herbal and Other Additives for Soap, pages 50–51), preserving the herbal benefits is less of a concern.

Since extracts are a more potent version of active ingredients, less is generally needed to gain the benefits and they are often added at trace in the soapmaking process. Some recipes in this book use tea to make the lye-water for an interesting twist; this is a different method than using extracts. (See Using Tea to Color Soap, page 65.)

All about Color

You can use many things to color your soap. The most common are food coloring (FD&C colorants), pigments and oxides, clays, and natural herbal infusions.

FD&C (Food, Drugs, and Cosmetics) are man-made colorants that are approved by the FDA for use in those three products. FD&C colorants can be found in ordinary foods (for example, farmed salmon and brightly colored candies), many brands of vitamins, and of course, cosmetics such as lipstick and eye shadow. Sold as LabColors, among other trade names, they produce vibrant colors that are fun, interesting, and varied. FD&C colorants are not considered natural, however. They are not used in any of the recipes in this book.

PIGMENTS AND OXIDES are a class of colorant that are either mined from the earth or manufactured in a lab. Because of impurities naturally found in products coming from the earth, pigments and oxides must be stringently purified to meet safety requirements regarding lead and other heavy metals. Many labs choose to bypass this process and instead manufacture pure colorants. Technically man-made, these colorants have the same chemical composition as mined ones, minus the heavy

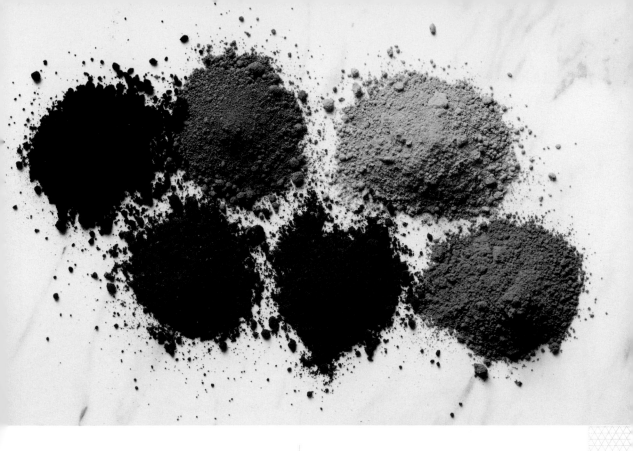

metals. Because of this, many people consider pigments and oxides as "natural" or "nature-identical." Pigments and oxides are light-fast and color-stable, meaning they do not fade and do not bleed in soap.

CLAYS are technically purified dirt. They are a natural raw material of mineral origin, composed of fine particles of silicates and many micro-minerals such as titanium, magnesium, copper, zinc, aluminum, calcium, potassium, nickel, manganese, lithium, sodium, and iron. Clays vary greatly based on where they come from, with the composition of the earth, the water, and the climate of a region changing properties such as color.

Clays in the United States are extracted from sites that are approved and controlled by the Bureau of Land Management and the United States Geological Survey. They are dried in the sun, ground to a fine consistency, and subjected to a heat and ozone gas process to kill microbial growth. Some clays are also sterilized using gamma irradiation. This is why utilizing actual dirt from your back yard is not a good idea; it will not have been purified to appropriate standards. Do not use craft clay, molding clay, or any other type that is not specifically designed for cosmetic use.

HERBAL OIL INFUSIONS are a common way of adding color to soap, even though they are technically not approved by the FDA for that purpose (see A Word from the FDA, page 44). The color imparted by some herbs does fade over time, so not all herbs can be considered colorfast. The result varies based on the herb used. See Herbal and Other Additives for Soap on pages 50–51 for more information.

Making Herbal Oil Infusions to Color Soap

Using natural herbs or colorants in your soap requires that you plan ahead, sometimes weeks in advance. Keep in mind that the natural color of the soapmaking oils and the color of your essential oil (used for scent) both color your soap; this is the color that provides the canvas from which you are starting. For example, an alkanet root infusion in cold-process soap normally creates a beautiful gray-purple-blue color. However, if you use orange 10x (very concentrated orange essential oil) with it, the color goes to an unattractive green.

Infusing herbs in oil is simple. It is best to use fully dried herbs to reduce the potential for contamination by yeast, mold, or bacteria in the final product. To achieve a strong color, most soapers use at least 2 tablespoons of herb for every 4 ounces of oil. I prefer to use a tablespoon of herb for every ounce. Use an oil with a long shelf life, such as jojoba oil or olive oil.

There are several methods for making herbal oil infusions. Infusions will keep in the refrigerator, so if you find that you like a particular one, make a larger batch so you'll have it on hand whenever you want to make soap. A reasonable amount might be a quarter to a half cup at a time.

Stovetop Oil Infusion

This method is significantly faster than doing a cold infusion and is the method suggested for the recipes in this book. Add the herbs and oil to the top pot of a double boiler and stir to cover the herbs. Bring the oil to medium heat (approximately 120°F [49°C]) then let the water in the bottom pot simmer for 4 hours, stirring the herbs every 20 minutes.

Record Your Data

Keeping good notes is key to reproducing great results, especially when working with something as crop-dependent as natural colorants. Here is some useful information to have:

» Name of herb/spice/tea/clay/colorant

» Date of infusion

» Batch number

» State of herbs (dry/fresh/whole/ground)

» Weather conditions

» Oils used

» Part of herb/spice/tea/clay used

» Infusion process

» Quantities of oils and infused product

» Storage conditions

» Date and process used to filter infusion

» Final quantity of oil

» Comments

Do not leave the stove unattended. If the oils get too hot (above 130–140°F [54–60°C]) the herbs will burn. This smells bad and turns your infusion brown.

Pour the infused oil through a fine-mesh strainer to remove most of the herbal matter, then filter it through a layer of cheesecloth to remove remaining larger particles or a coffee filter for fine particles. Funnel the colored oil into clean bottles and store in the refrigerator.

ALTERNATE METHOD: Add dried herbs to a heat-sealable teabag, filling the bag just halfway full. (You want them to have room for the oil to mix in.) Put the bag into the oil in

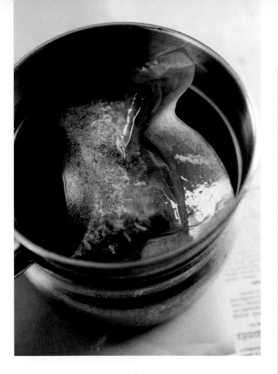

A HEAT-SEALABLE teabag is a convenient way to infuse herbs into oil.

Storing Infused Oils

Most of the recipes in this book call for just a few teaspoons of infused oil, but it makes sense to make at least a tablespoon or two for any given recipe, as it's hard to work with smaller amounts. You can keep the leftover oil for use in other batches, so if you soap a lot, it might make sense to scale up the amounts to a quarter cup or more so that you have some on hand when you need it.

No matter what your infusion method, store infused oils in the refrigerator to help prevent mold and bacterial growth caused by any bits of herb left after straining. You might be tempted to add vitamin E oil, rosemary oil extract, or grapefruit seed extract as a preservative, but while these are effective antioxidants, they are not preservatives. Using them will protect against rancidity but will not prevent mold or bacteria from forming. Use all infused oils within 6 months.

Synthetic preservatives for oil-based formulas — for example, LiquaPar oil, LiquaPar Optima, LiquaPar PE, and Phenonip — are available, but I have never found it necessary to use them. The risk of mold is slight to begin with and refrigeration is effective.

a double boiler or, if doing several infusions at once, put each bag in a separate canning jar with oil. Make sure the oil comes close to reaching the lid. Screw the lid on tight. Place the jars in a hot-water bath on medium heat for 4 hours, never leaving the setup unattended.

Cold Oil Infusion

Add the herbs to a small glass jar and cover them with oil. Seal the jar and set it aside for 4 to 6 weeks, checking weekly to ensure there is no mold on the herbs or condensation forming on the underside of the lid. If you do find any moisture, wipe the lid with rubbing alcohol and a clean paper towel. When the steeping period is over, filter the oil through a fine-mesh strainer and then through a layer of cheesecloth or a coffee filter to remove any last remnants.

Using Clay to Color Soap

When working with clays in cold-process soap, it is important to take into account their effect on the soaping process. Clays are added as powders, so they will absorb moisture, either while you are mixing them or during the curing period. The addition of clay can accelerate trace, meaning you have to be ready to pour it in the molds immediately. It also limits your ability to work with patterns and designs.

Different clays have varying levels of absorption, so always try a small test batch prior to making a big batch of a clay soap.

Adding Clay

There are two ways to incorporate clay easily and (mostly) effortlessly into your cold-process soap. For this book, all of the clays are used with the following method.

Using a mini mixer, combine the required amounts of clay and water 4 hours in advance of starting your recipe. Generally, a ratio of 3 parts of water to 1 part of clay works well. If the clay absorbs too much water, add more water until the mixture remains liquid (strive for a consistency somewhere between cake batter and fudge). Add this slurry to your soap before you add your essential oil, and mix it in well.

You can also add the clay directly to the water before mixing in the lye. The heat reaction from the lye-water will produce a deeper color than will adding the clay at thin trace, so if utilizing this method, start with half the clay you were planning to use.

With this method, any small amount of grit or sand in the clay will fall to the bottom of your mixture, so prior to adding the lye-water and clay solution to your soap, strain it through a stainless steel strainer lined with a coffee filter to remove the undissolved grit. Be prepared, though; your batch may still accelerate.

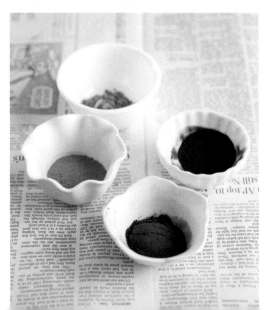

Herbal and Other Additives for Soap

YELLOW/GREEN

Olive leaf powder

● **Yellow/green**
2 tsp powder per pound of soap. Will fade with exposure to light.

Comfrey powder

● **Light green**
2 tsp powder per pound of soap. Gel phase enhances the color. Will fade substantially with exposure to light.

Nettle leaf powder

● **Green**
2 tsp powder per pound of soap. Beautiful green color will fade with exposure to light, but is more stable than some other natural greens.

Spirulina powder

● **Deep green**
2 tsp powder per pound of soap. Color is enhanced by a hot gel phase, but will fade substantially with exposure to light.

Indigo powder

- **Blue/gray**
2 tsp powder per pound of soap. Can be added as a dispersed powder (shown in photo on page 53) or added directly to hot lye-water before combining oils.

Alkanet root powder

- **Purple/gray**
2 tsp powder per pound of soap. Can be used as an infusion or dispersed powder. Infusion will fade over time; dispersed powder is more color stable.

Orange essential oil

- **Pale yellow**
0.8 oz essential oil per pound of soap. Will fade with exposure to light.

Annatto

- **Bright orange**
2 tsp infusion per pound of soap. Will fade somewhat with exposure to light, but a stronger infusion will help it hold its color.

Paprika

- **Red/orange**
2 tsp powder per pound of soap. Can also be infused and added at 4 tsp infusion per pound of soap. Gives a speckled appearance; color will leach out from spots over time.

Rose clay

- **Rosy pink**
2 tsp powder per pound of soap. Disperse in distilled water instead of oil. Holds color nicely and will not fade.

Madder root powder

- **Dark red**
2 tsp powder per pound of soap. Can be added as a dispersed powder or infused.

Yarrow powder

- **Yellow/tan**
2 tsp powder per pound of soap. Dispersed powder can be added at trace, or the dry powder can be infused into lye-water to create a more yellow hue.

Cocoa powder

- **Rich brown**
2 tsp powder per pound of soap. Gel phase enhances the color, as does exposure to air.

FOR THE SOAPS featured on the following pages, all powdered additives were dispersed at a ratio of 1 part powder: 3 parts oil. (For infusion directions, see page 48.) The colorants were added at trace and went through gel phase. The usage rates listed above represent the color shown in the photos on the next two pages; increase or decrease the amount of colorant used to achieve your desired color. Note that some of the soaps look grainy initially but the color evens out over time.

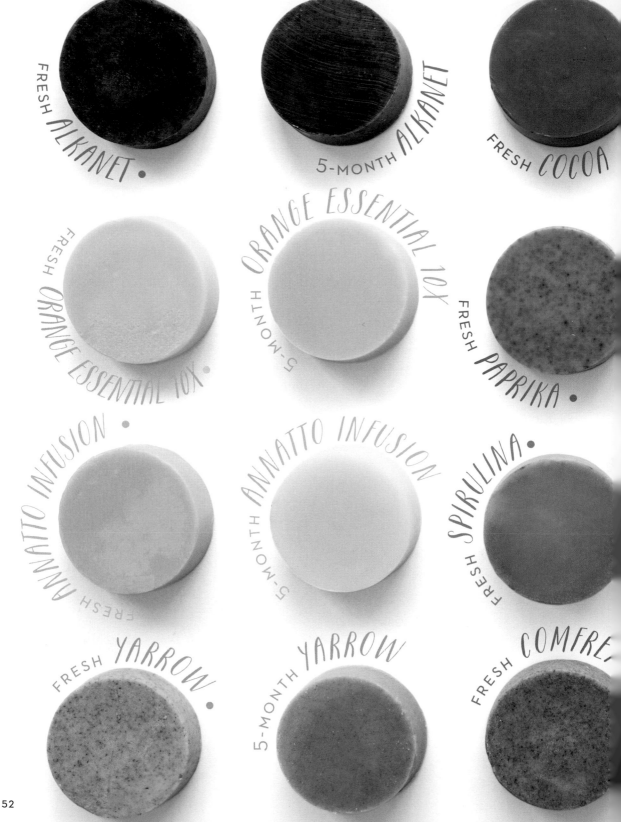

FRESH ALKANET •

5-MONTH ALKANET

FRESH COCOA

FRESH ORANGE ESSENTIAL 10X •

ORANGE ESSENTIAL 10X

5-MONTH

FRESH PAPRIKA •

FRESH ANNATTO INFUSION •

5-MONTH ANNATTO INFUSION

FRESH SPIRULINA •

FRESH YARROW •

5-MONTH YARROW

FRESH COMFRE

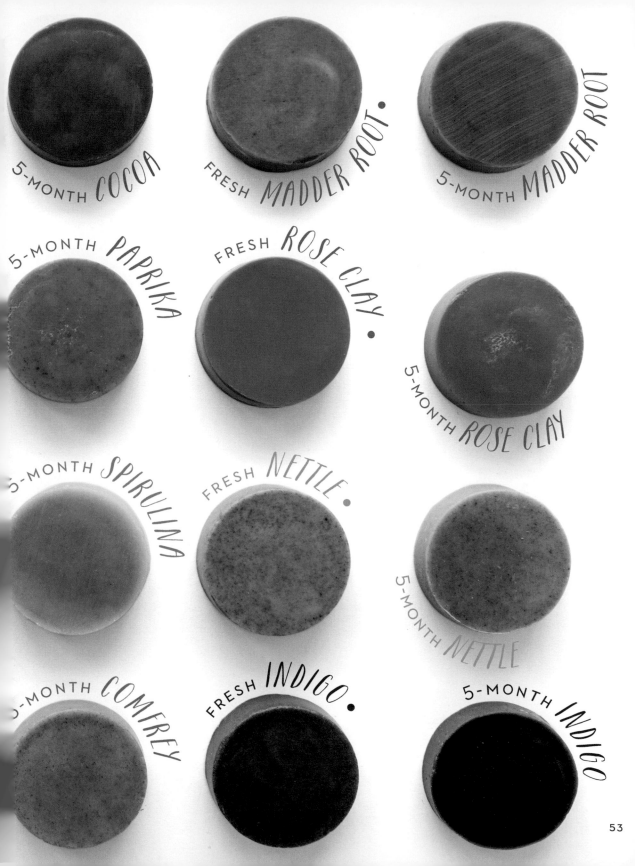

5-MONTH *COCOA*

FRESH *MADDER ROOT* •

5-MONTH *MADDER ROOT*

5-MONTH *PAPRIKA*

FRESH *ROSE CLAY* •

5-MONTH *ROSE CLAY*

5-MONTH *SPIRULINA*

FRESH *NETTLE* •

5-MONTH *NETTLE*

5-MONTH *COMFREY*

FRESH *INDIGO* •

5-MONTH *INDIGO*

53

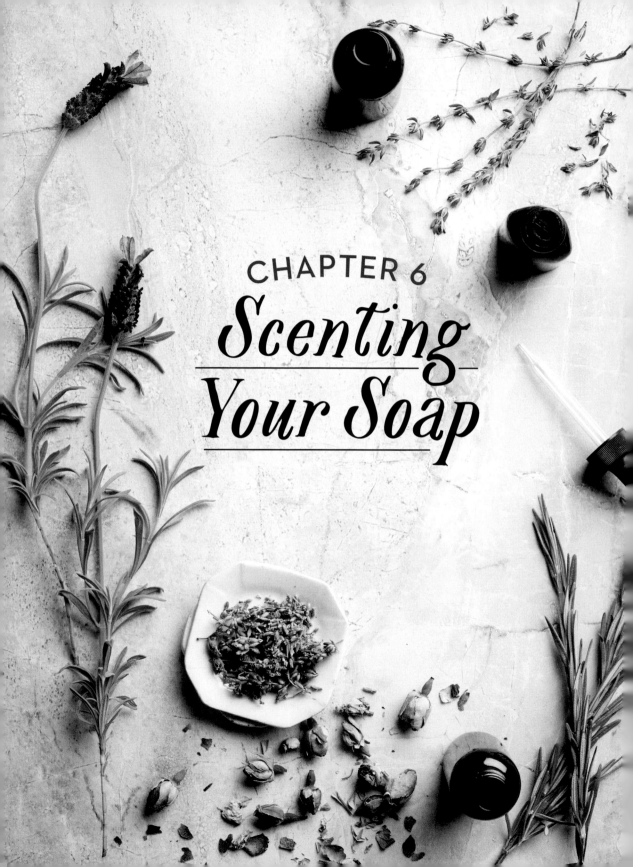

CHAPTER 6

Scenting Your Soap

Y OU CAN CREATE any type of fragrance you can think of using fragrance oils. Though they mimic floral, spicy, or fruity scents, fragrance oils are synthetic compounds created in labs. They are typically proprietary blends made by different companies. Fragrance oils can be used to scent soap when there is no natural alternative, such as cherry or chocolate.

Because they are made with a consistent formula, fragrance oils always smell the same. They are not considered natural, although you can buy, for example, both lavender fragrance oil and lavender essential oil. (See What Are "Nature-Identical" Oils?, page 57.) Because they are not considered natural, this book does not use any synthetic fragrance oils.

About Essential Oils

Essential oils are derived directly from the stems, leaves, bark, or petals of plants and trees. They can be extracted in a variety of ways, though the most common method is by steam distillation, a process that forces steam through the plant matter, releasing the oil, which is then separated from the water. The resulting oil is called "essential oil" and the water is called a "hydrosol." This type of extraction is commonly done with oilier or denser plant matter, such as citrus peel, bay laurel, and cedarwood.

Essential oils typically have a shorter shelf life than fragrance oils and may smell different from batch to batch, as the crops from which they are made will be different every year. Generally, the more precious the ingredient, the higher the price of the oil.

Other types of essential oil distillations are solvent extraction, enfleurage, and CO_2 extraction. Enfleurage infuses odorless, solid fats with plant matter to capture the fragrance. It is expensive and inefficient, but is the best option for delicate plants whose fragrance would be destroyed by steam distillation. CO_2 extraction sometimes replaces enfleurage as a more modern method for extracting the essential oil out of delicate plants. Solvent extraction results in both an essential oil and an almost solid, waxy substance called a "concrete."

The more precious essential oils are expensive to use in soap. If you want to use an exotic essential oil, such as rose essential oil or jasmine concrete, consider making rebatch soap and adding the essential oil at the end to preserve the oil's precious qualities and scent.

Because this book focuses on natural ingredients, these recipes use only all-natural, traditionally distilled essential oils.

Scenting with Essential Oils

Scenting is typically the last step before pouring soap into molds, as many essential oils accelerate trace. When scenting with essential oils, take the following factors into account.

SAFETY. Essential oils are powerful. Not all of them are recommended for use by pregnant women, for example. Thoroughly research any essential oil or essential oil blend you want to craft with before making soap with it.

Many essential oils are flammable, so store them in a cool place and keep out of sunlight. Do not store them in plastic, which will deteriorate over time. Wear gloves when working with essential oils; they can degrade fingernail polish, as well as paint and wood finishes.

PURITY. Because essential oils can be expensive, unscrupulous vendors may add synthetic fragrance components or diluents to their products to stretch them and make more money. Only buy from established vendors that do gas chromatography (GC) or mass spectrometry (MS) checks on their oils to test for purity.

STABILITY. Essential oils can be delicate. The environment of soapmaking, with a pH of up to 14, is often too harsh for a particular essential oil to survive. Some essential oils, such as volatile citrus oils, never last in cold-process soap.

Soaping with some essential oils takes extra measures, such as blending them with an anchor scent, which is a scent of a similar nature that does last in soap. For example, you can combine volatile lime essential oil with sturdier lemongrass essential oil to create a scent that remains in the final bars. You can also use a redistilled oil such as orange 5x or orange 10x; this means that the essential oil has been distilled multiple times to make it more potent.

Blending Essential Oils

Essential oils are volatile and evaporate quickly. Blending them can improve their shelf life and help emphasize individual notes. Blending essential oils to create signature scents is fun and easy. It is also an art. What smells great to one person may not be attractive to another.

Before blending, you should understand the chemistry of your oils. Blending essential oils typically takes into account top, middle, and base or bottom notes, all of which appear in a successful blend. Normally, top notes are the lighter notes that tend to evaporate quickly. They often form your first impression of a perfume and are typically citrus notes such as lemon and lemongrass; peppermint is another.

Middle notes comprise the heart or the main body of a perfume. They emerge as the top notes start to waft off. These fragrances are more mellow and are often floral in nature. Examples are lavender, chamomile, and ylang ylang.

Base notes hold the entire perfume together. They bring depth and often boost the strength of a blend. Typically these rich, deep notes — think patchouli and sandalwood — are often not perceived until 30 minutes after scent application.

When blending, consider the overall fragrance. A bright citrus scent will dissipate quickly, so consider adding a middle or an anchoring base note like Egyptian geranium to give the blend more depth. A deeper note like patchouli could be easily lightened up with a sweet floral or bright citrus.

A Quick How-To

Blending essential oils is as simple as planning your blend and trying a few options. Keep ample notes so you remember what you like. Remember, a blend will smell differently after an hour than it does when first mixed. Here's how to start:

1. Mix a few drops each of the desired essential oils in a small glass container. To fully appreciate the scent, dip a strip of paper into the oils and sniff it.

2. Smell the paper a few times over the next hour, noting how the scent changes as the higher top notes dissipate and the base notes begin to show through.

3. Once you have a blend or two that smell great, test them in soap. A 1-pound batch of soap can be split into four containers and each scented with a different essential oil blend. For 4 ounces of soap, add up to 0.125 ounce of essential oil.

Making a small sample batch will allow you to get a feel for how the essential oil blend holds up in soap after curing and what the final product will smell like without as much investment as a large batch.

SAFE DILUTION RATES

(according to the National Association for Holistic Aromatherapy)

For infants and young children:	
DILUTION	DROPS OF ESSENTIAL OIL PER OUNCE OF CARRIER
0.5–1%	3–6

For adults:	
DILUTION	DROPS OF ESSENTIAL OIL PER OUNCE OF CARRIER
0.5–1%	3–6
2.5%	15
3%	20
5%	30
10%	60

What Are "Nature-Identical" Oils?

Fragrance oils are created from a blend of "aroma chemicals" — individual molecules that contain single fragrance notes — suspended in a carrier liquid. Aroma chemicals can be synthetic, natural, or nature-identical.

Synthetic fragrance oils are specifically created to be aromatically pleasing. The chemical compound may not be found in nature, but can still produce a distinct, recognizable smell. For example, the scent of watermelon cannot be extracted from the actual fruit, but the artificial version is instantly recognizable. Other scents in this category include banana, cherry, and chocolate, not to mention cupcake, bubblegum, and fruit punch.

A natural-aroma chemical is derived directly from a plant, but the specific scent molecule is isolated from the other components of the plant. This single-molecule product differs from an essential oil, which has a more complex profile. A natural-aroma chemical does not have the same aromatherapy effects as its essential oil counterpart, as it does not contain the full spectrum of components that make up an essential oil.

A nature-identical fragrance oil is a chemical replica of an essential oil that is created in a lab. For example, a nature-identical lavender fragrance does not necessarily start with lavender buds, but it contains the exact same blend of chemicals that are found in real lavender oil. Some soapers do not consider nature-identical fragrance oils to be "natural," but might be hard pressed to explain what the difference is. Molecules are molecules: nature-identical oils have the same range of components as essential oils and cannot be distinguished from them by their chemical structure. As with many ingredients, it comes down to an individual choice to use them or not.

Safety Guidelines

Essential oils are concentrated and can cause skin irritation when used straight. Please use safety guidelines and follow standard dilution guidelines.

Use stainless steel or glass bowls and mixing utensils. Do not use plastic unless it is a chemical-resistant plastic. Essential oils can eat through soft plastics and ruin work surfaces.

Some essential oils can cause adverse skin reactions such as irritation, dermal sensitization, and even photosensitization, and should be avoided (see Not for Soaping on facing page). If exposure to oils causes any of the mentioned reactions, remove contaminated clothing and wash exposed area with soapy water. If any essential oils come in contact with eyes, flush eyes with water for a minimum of 10 to 20 minutes. If necessary, seek medical attention.

If ingested, do not induce vomiting. Rinse your mouth with water and seek immediate assistance from your local poison center or hospital.

If pregnant, follow all safety guidelines and consult with your physician.

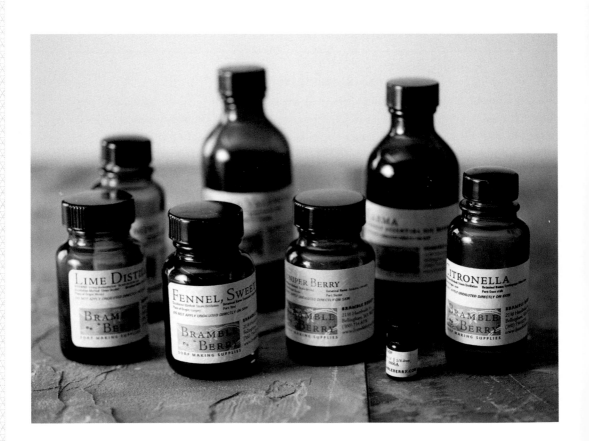

Not for Soaping

Not all essential oils are safe to use in soap. Some produce side effects such as skin irritation and allergic reactions. Always research the essential oil you are using before crafting with it. These are some essential oils that have safety warnings:

- » Bitter almond
- » Boldo
- » Cade
- » Calamus
- » Camphor (yellow)
- » Costus root
- » Elecampane oil
- » Fig leaf absolute
- » Goosefoot
- » Horseradish
- » Melissa

- » Mugwort
- » Mustard
- » Pennyroyal
- » Rue
- » Sassafras
- » Savin
- » Tansy
- » Thuja
- » Wintergreen
- » Wormseed
- » Wormwood

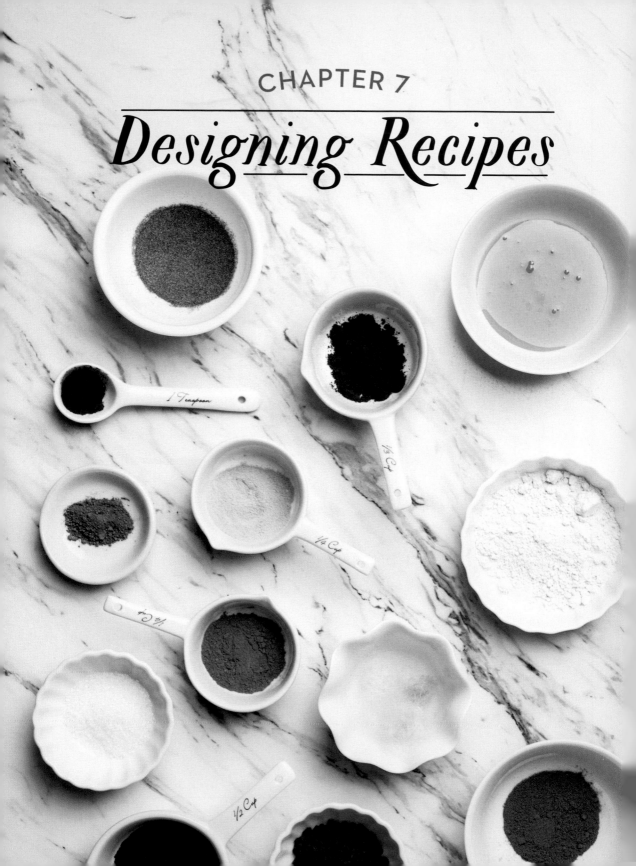

CHAPTER 7

Designing Recipes

WHAT MAKES A GREAT SOAP recipe is intensely personal. Some people prefer plenty of lather, but those with hard water have a difficult time getting any lather unless a particular blend of oils is used. Others prefer a slick conditioning bar or a lot of exfoliation in their soap.

Designing your own recipes also means your favorite ingredient can make an appearance in all your products, or you can try out some new additives to help improve your skin's look and feel. You can increase the amount of butters to provide more moisture to dry skin, or use aloe vera, essential oils, and other plant extracts for homeopathic effects. You can design a mild cleansing bar for use on children or create a shampoo bar for cleaning hair.

Crafting Your Own Recipes

Designing new recipes can be exciting and a little intimidating, but don't worry, you don't need to reinvent the wheel to create your own versions. Before you dive in, though, become familiar with a few established recipes. Choose ones that sound good, with ingredients that you and your skin will like. Once you have some experience, trying variations with a tried-and-true recipe is a great place to start creating your own recipes.

Modifying existing recipes with different oils and extracts will give you the confidence to use common guidelines and oil properties to create your soap from scratch. The general rule of thumb is to replace oils with similar oils; that is, replace solid oils with other solids, and liquid oils with other liquids. For example, olive oil is a good substitute for canola oil, but cocoa butter is not. Read chapter 5 to learn about usage rates for individual oils.

The colors and essential oils may also be swapped out, but make sure to find out how a new ingredient performs in cold-process soap before you make a whole batch. Some essential oils will accelerate trace, for instance, and some colors morph or just disappear.

The best way to determine how a new recipe will turn out is to do a small test batch, wait the full 4 to 6 weeks for a cure time, and evaluate it. As with most things, practice makes perfect — pretty soon, you'll be formulating with confidence and achieving the bars you want each and every time.

CAUTION: If you change any of the oils in a recipe, you *must* run it through a lye calculator again to ensure the correct amount of lye is used. In fact, whenever you modify a recipe in any way, always run it through a lye calculator, as the water and lye values can change with even small adjustments. Getting the lye-water and oil proportions are critical to getting your soap to trace and cure properly.

Making That Special Soap

Here are some additional tips for designing recipes with specific properties.

For a luxurious bar for silky skin

» Pile on the nourishing oils (see chapter 4). These include avocado oil, meadowfoam oil, and butters. You can also add luxurious oils such as argan oil (up to 10 percent) and hemp-seed oil (less than 20 percent).

Resizing Recipes

All of the recipes in this book list the weight of each ingredient and the percentage of the total oil content. Whether you are increasing or decreasing the original recipes, the ratio of lye, oils, and liquid must remain the same. To do something simple like make a double batch, just multiply all of the ingredient amounts by 2 or run the recipe through a lye calculator using the increased amounts. To cut the recipe in half, simply divide the amount of each needed ingredient by 2. It's always a good idea to double-check even simple math with a lye calculator.

» Increase the superfat. Leaving some unsaponified oils in your soap increases the nourishing, moisturizing properties.

» Use additives, such as silk or some clays, to increase the silky feeling of the final lather in the bar (see chapter 5).

For a bar with lots of lather

» Castor oil is great for adding some much-needed bubbles to your soap. However, adding more than 4 to 7 percent can create a sticky bar of soap, the opposite of what you are trying to design. For lather improvements, keep this additive at 3 percent or below.

» Cut back that superfat. If your soap is superfatted higher than 8 percent, all those free-floating oils can kill lather.

» A half teaspoon of sugar per pound of soap added to your lye-water can help your bar lather up. Using liquids such as beer, fruit juices, and wine that contain sugar also boosts bubbles.

» Palm oil and coconut oil work synergistically together to produce thick lather. When used on their own, the bubbles are not as large or stable.

» Decrease oils that don't add to lather, such as avocado oil and shea butter.

For a hard bar

» Use more hard (solid at room temperature) oils in your recipe. These include palm oil, coconut oil, cocoa butter, and shea butter.

» Common table salt will create harder soap. Add it at a rate of 1/2 teaspoon per pound of oil in a recipe. Add the salt to the water first and stir well to dissolve it before adding the lye.

» Sodium lactate is a popular soaping ingredient that creates a shiny, hard bar of soap. Add it at a rate of 1 teaspoon per pound of oils to your lye-water. As a bonus, it cuts unmolding time roughly in half.

» Beeswax is a natural hardening agent. You can use it up to 3 percent in your recipe, but you must soap at a higher temperature (145°F [63°C] and above) to keep it from hardening. Using too much beeswax can decrease lather.

» Do a water discount. This means using 10–15 percent less water than the recipe calls for. This is a more advanced technique (see What Is a Water Discount? on the facing page) and should only be attempted after many successful soap batches.

What a Difference the Oil Makes

Oils at room temperature can be liquid (olive oil) or solid (coconut oil), but it is difficult to generalize final bar properties from that state. For example, you would probably assume that oils that are solid at room temperature produce a harder bar of soap. This assumption is correct, but it is the only thing you can assume when formulating recipes. For example, coconut oil produces amazing lather, but cocoa butter, which is also solid at room temperature, does not have great lather when used on its own. This is why it is important to find a mixture of oils that produce the final end result you want.

Oils work synergistically to produce a great bar of soap. For example, although shea butter adds to the moisturizing and conditioning properties of a soap, if you use it at 100 percent, the bar will not lather well. If you combine it with coconut oil, however, it will produce a bar that balances the skin-care properties of shea butter with a wonderful lather.

To illustrate this further, here are three recipes that use different quantities of olive, coconut, and palm oil. Olive oil contributes a small lather with conditioning properties; it is good for sensitive skin. Coconut oil creates large lather, has good cleansing properties, and adds to bar hardness. Palm oil stabilizes the lather and contributes cleansing and bar hardness.

Recipe 1:
33% olive + 33% coconut + 34% palm

» With high palm and high coconut percentages, this soap will cure into hard bars with excellent cleansing and lather abilities. The olive oil will provide some moisturizing and conditioning properties but not enough to offset the cleansing ability of the coconut and palm. At a 5% superfat, this bar will possess large, copious bubbles, but may feel slightly drying to some skin types.

Recipe 2:
50% olive + 25% coconut + 25% palm

» This recipe nicely balances the olive oil's superior conditioning and moisturizing abilities. The coconut oil and palm oil contribute to bar stability, lather, and bar hardness. At a 5% superfat, this bar will have medium-sized bubbles that last and will leave skin feeling clean but not dry.

What Is a Water Discount?

Water discounting is an advanced technique that involves holding back some of the liquid (usually water) that is mixed with the lye in the beginning. Some soapers do it on purpose to make their soap cure faster and produce harder bars that won't shrink over time as excess moisture evaporates. Using less water means that the recipe will trace faster, which is why this is an advanced technique.

Note that when utilizing a water discount specifically to add tea or another ingredient at the end of the soapmaking process, you will not receive the benefits (curing faster, harder bars) described, because you end up adding the same amount of water in the end.

Recipe 3:
90% olive + 5% coconut + 5% palm

» Because this soap is primarily olive oil, it will have small lather and be extremely moisturizing and conditioning. The coconut and palm will provide some bar hardness and lather stability, but the final bar will still have a smooth, small lather and will be prone to developing a layer of goo in a wet environment. At a 5% superfat, this bar will have small, slick bubbles that leave the skin feeling clean and even.

See chapter 4 to learn about the properties and SAP values of specific oils.

Using Other Liquids

You can use liquids other than water to make your lye solution. Coffee, tea, milk, beer, and wine can add interest and skin-loving properties, plus they have great marketing value on the label, if you are selling your products. It's important to prepare each liquid appropriately prior to adding the lye, as misuse can not only ruin your soap, but also be dangerous during the process.

Coffee and Tea

Caffeine constricts blood vessels and may temporarily help to even out skin tones, so coffee and teas that contain caffeine are thought to help reduce skin redness. Numerous cellulite-reducing products on the marketplace utilize caffeine.

Coffee, both ground and brewed, absorbs odors, so soap that contains some coffee, either brewed or ground, is ideal for removing pungent odors from hands. Liquid coffee also tints the soap a rich brown; however, you probably won't detect much, if any, lingering coffee scent due to the saponification process.

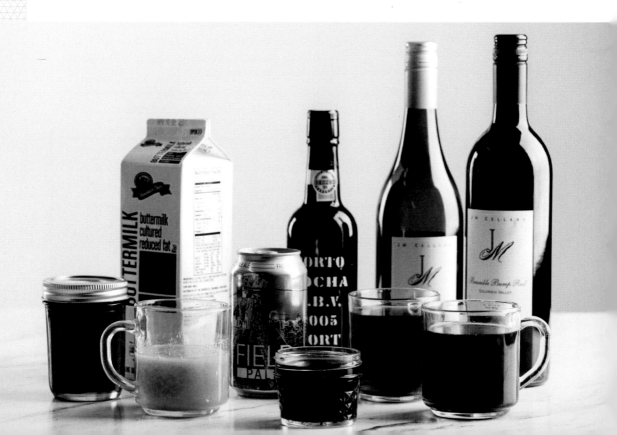

Using Tea to Color Soap

Teas do not work well on their own as colorants. The tannins in the tea react with the lye solution by turning dark or by completely leaching out and leaving no final color. If the tea has caffeine in it, it usually will turn brown in soap, but not always a pleasing shade. Black tea has the highest level of caffeine and produces the darkest color.

The best way to add tea, if you are trying to maintain color, is to make a strong slurry of tea, freeze the tea in ice cube trays, water discount with your lye (see What Is a Water Discount? on page 63) and then add the ice cubes (factoring in the water discount) after you add the scent. This will help preserve some of the colorant but not all of it.

Rooibos and herbal teas can be prepared this way. Since they do not contain caffeine, they do maintain some color. Rooibos turns a red/brown color in soaps, for example.

With teas, the resulting color is always brown or olive green. Even red elderflower tea, for example, will turn brown during saponification. Green tea can initially color soap a lovely green, though the final soap turns brown as it cures. Bergamot-based teas give soap a creamy color and, depending on the strength of the infusion, may impart a faint bergamot scent after saponification. Minty teas also give soap a brown, creamy color and the aroma tends to linger a bit.

When using coffee or tea in place of water, chill it to nearly ice-cold before adding the lye, to prevent it from scorching (this smells awful!). Use the coffee/tea, brewed to normal strength, just as you would water, replacing it in any recipe in the amount specified for the water.

Alcoholic or Carbonated Beverages

Beer and wine add a few positive attributes to soap but offer an interesting soaping challenge. They contain fantastic antioxidants, and the natural sugars increase lather. The color of the alcohol greatly affects the final appearance of the soap. A dark merlot will result in a much darker final bar than a soap made using a chardonnay, so keep that in mind when designing a recipe around a color palette. The end results are worth the extra time needed to add the alcohol.

Beer, wine, and champagne require some additional preparation, so leave extra time when using them and follow safety procedures even more scrupulously than usual. It is critical to boil off the carbonation and alcohol from these liquids before using them in soap, or a volcanic eruption may occur when you add the lye. To do this, boil the liquid uncovered for 10 to 15 minutes, then put it in the fridge, uncovered, and leave it for 24 hours. Boiling reduces the volume, so you need to start with roughly twice the amount of liquid as the recipe calls for.

Beverages that have a high alcohol and/or sugar content become extremely hot when lye is added to them. Both alcohol and other clear liquids, such as teas, work best when chilled, and it's important to add the lye slowly to the cooled liquid. This helps keep the overall soap temperature down, preserves a more neutral color, and helps give the time you may need to work with a more intricate recipe.

Juices and Purees

Fruit and vegetable juices and purees are packed full of nourishing vitamins, minerals, and beautiful natural colors. Vitamins A, B_6, and C are found in many vegetables and fruits, along with copious amounts of antioxidants that fight free radicals. Carrots, tomatoes, and cucumber skins can provide beautiful color in soaps, though be aware that soaps colored with purees will fade over time. If you're selling your soap, adding purees adds flair to your label and sets your product apart from the competition.

When adding juices to soap, always add the lye directly to chilled juice. Add a liquid puree at thin trace or as a portion of the water phase. It is important to add the juice or puree with the lye-water or at thin trace so that the pH of the mixture is high enough to kill off any possibility of mold or bacteria in the fruit. Whenever possible, use pure fruit juices that you have prepared yourself.

Purees must be finely ground; never use chunks of fruit or vegetable in soap. Larger pieces of fruit or vegetables will eventually mold or cause a discoloring "halo" effect. You can use pure fruit juice in place of all or part of the liquid/water portion of your recipe. The puree can be added at thin trace or watered down and used as all or a portion of the lye-water. Purees and fruit juices do not add scent to the soap.

Many purees or fruit juices do go brown or fade over time. There are some exceptions — carrot juice and pumpkin puree, for example — that keep their color for some time, but for the most part, purees and fruit juices are not ideal coloring agents. To help the colors last, store soaps in a dark place. The amount of time the color will remain in the soap varies with the additive, with greens typically being the shortest-lived before turning brown. The shelf life of soap made with fresh veggie or fruit juices and purees is about one year, even if the color fades before that time.

Milk

Cleopatra is said to have bathed in donkey milk daily to keep her skin radiant and youthful. While it is no longer common to bathe in a tub full of milk, milk soaps are increasingly popular for their skin benefits. All milks (nut and animal) contain skin-loving fats and proteins. Some, such as goat milk, contain lactic acid, which encourages skin cell turnover and smoother skin. Milk soaps tend to have rich, creamy lathers and leave the skin feeling soft from the excess fats.

When buying milks, look for ingredients without additives, such as thickeners or sugars. Thickeners (guar gum is a common one) can significantly speed up trace and make it difficult to complete intricate designs. Added sugars in milk will cause excess heat to form, which can result in the soap puffing out of the mold like a soufflé, as well as discoloration.

Soaping with milk requires a somewhat different process. Milk that becomes too hot from the lye will scorch, causing discoloration and a foul odor, so for best results, work with frozen or slightly thawed (slushy) milk. The more slowly you add the lye to the frozen milk, the less chance you have for discoloration and scorching. Start with about 1 tablespoon of lye, sprinkle it on the cubes or slush, stir until dissolved (it will melt the ice), and repeat 1 tablespoon at a time until all the lye has been added. Placing the lye-water container into a cold-water or ice-water bath will also help to keep it from getting too hot.

What Are INS Numbers?

Some new soapers like to use INS numbers. INS numbers refer to a numerical value that describes the properties an oil will have when reacted with sodium hydroxide to make bar soap. It relates to the degree of unsaturation and molecular weight of the oil. The theory was developed in the 1930s and over time, the meaning of acronym has been lost. Some people believe INS stands for Iodine iN Soap.

The iodine value is an old-fashioned way of determining the level of saturated versus unsaturated fats in various oils. Oils with more saturated fats dissolve less iodine, have lower iodine values, and give harder soap. Oils with more unsaturated fats dissolve more iodine, have higher iodine values, and give a softer soap.

An INS number is supposed to tell at a glance how an oil will perform in terms of hardness, conditioning, lather, and cleansing. Finding the perfect balance of oils is the holy grail of soapmaking; there would be no more thinking about how to design the best recipe for conditioning ability that also lathers well. In reality, it doesn't quite work that way.

For one thing, INS numbers cannot accommodate the variations among oils from crop to crop. Depending on where an oil is grown, how it is harvested, and how the climate changed from one batch to the next, its properties for making soap will be slightly different (really, truly!).

For another, soap recipes turn out differently depending on a variety of factors, such as where you are soaping. Soaping in a hot, dry room can produce different results than soaping in a cold, humid garage or basement. The actual bars of soap also behave differently depending on how you use them (note the difference when using hard water versus soft, for instance). Soaps also lather differently depending on the temperature of the water — the warmer the water, the better the lather.

In theory, a perfect bar of soap would result from a recipe with an INS number of 160, based on the INS numbers of all the oils used. In practice, however, a recipe using 100 percent cocoa butter, which has almost a perfect INS number, would produce slimy bars that don't lather and leave a sticky feel when rinsed off. Learn to create a great bar based on the properties the oils give to the bar, rather than relying on the imprecise method of INS numbers for determining your formulas.

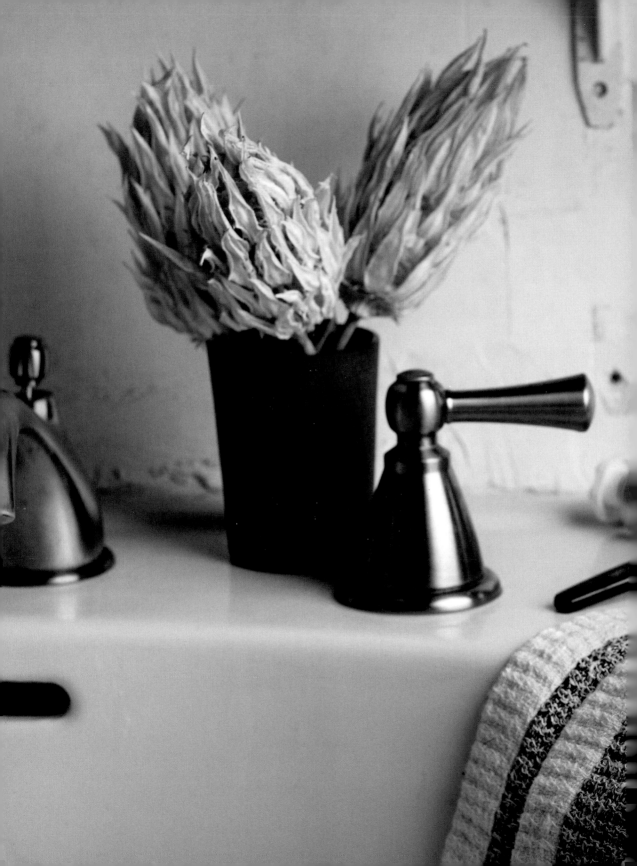

CHAPTER 8

All about Simplicity

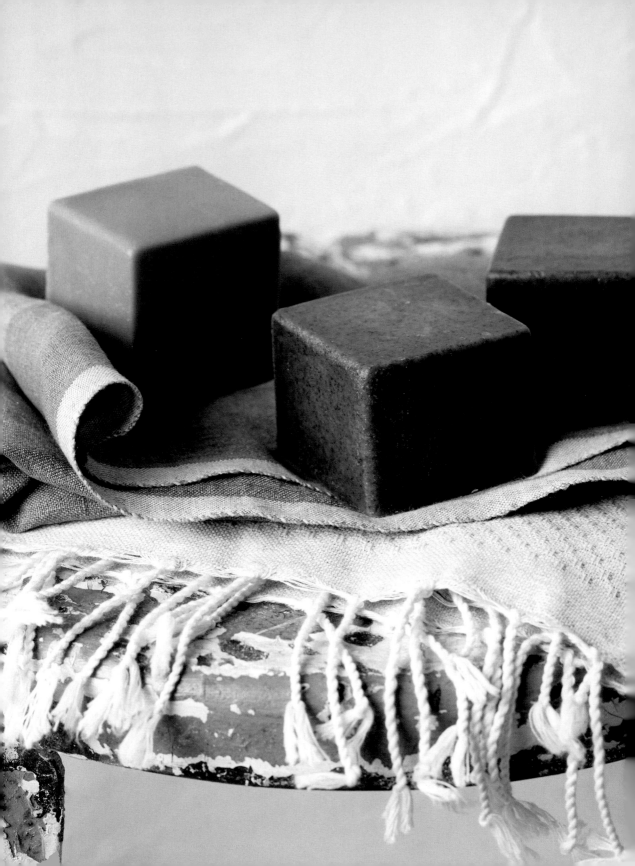

Comfrey & Spirulina
MULTICOLORED CUBES

Makes 9 bars

Spirulina is a dark-green algae that grows in lakes. It is rich in essential fatty acids, such as Omega-3s, -6s, and -9s, that are great for the skin. Comfrey leaves contain allantoin, which is said to protect the skin and promote new cell growth. The addition of refreshing rosemary and peppermint essential oils cools the skin and awakens the mind.

Mold and Special Tools

» 9-bar silicone cube mold
» Heating pad

Lye-Water Amounts

5.1 ounces lye (5% superfat)
11.5 ounces distilled water
2 teaspoons sodium lactate (optional)

Oil Amounts

8.5 ounces palm oil (23%)
9.2 ounces coconut oil (25%)
1.9 ounces avocado butter (5%)
11.1 ounces olive oil pure (30%)
0.7 ounce castor oil (2%)
5.6 ounces rice bran oil (15%)

Essential Oil Blend

1.1 ounces rosemary essential oil
0.3 ounce peppermint essential oil, 2nd distill

Colorant and Additive Amounts

1 tablespoon comfrey powder dispersed into 1 tablespoon rice bran oil

1 teaspoon spirulina powder dispersed into 1 tablespoon rice bran oil

1 teaspoon rose clay dispersed into 1 tablespoon distilled water

1 teaspoon alkanet root powder dispersed into 1 tablespoon rice bran oil

Note: This mold creates beautiful bars, but it can be tricky to remove them if sodium lactate is not included.

Safe Soaping!

Wear proper safety gear the whole time.

Work in a well-ventilated space.

No distractions (keep kids and pets away).

MAKE THE SOAP MIXTURE

1. Add the lye to the water (never the other way around) and stir gently until all of the lye is dissolved. If using sodium lactate, add it to the lye-water and stir to combine. Set aside until clear.

2. Melt the palm oil in its original container, mix it thoroughly, and measure into a bowl large enough to hold all of the oils and the lye-water with room to mix them. Melt and measure the coconut oil and add it to the bowl. Add the avocado butter to the hot oils and stir until melted. If needed, heat the oils further until the butter is melted. Add the olive oil pure, castor oil, and rice bran oil.

3. When both the oils and the lye-water are between 110° and 120°F (43–49°C), add the lye-water to the oils, pouring it over a spatula or the shaft of the stick blender to minimize air bubbles. Tap the blades a couple of times against the bottom of the bowl to release any trapped air. *Do not turn on the stick blender until it is fully immersed.* Stick-blend for 20 seconds, or until very light trace is achieved.

MIX AND POUR

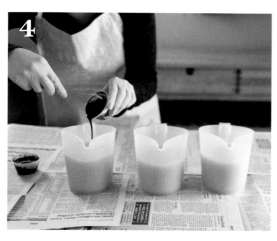

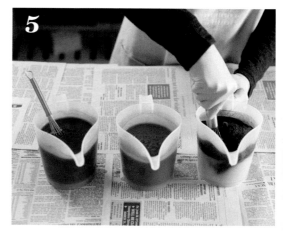

4. Divide the soap into three equal parts and add the full amount of each colorant as follows.
   » Container A: Comfrey and spirulina
   » Container B: Rose clay
   » Container C: Alkanet root

5. Divide the essential oil evenly among the containers, and whisk to combine the colorant and the essential oil.

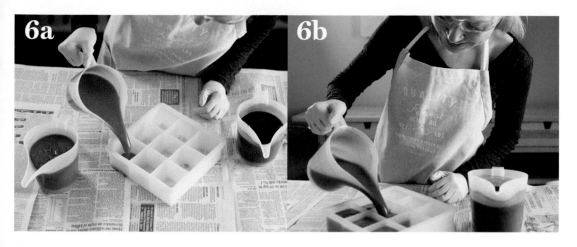

6. Pour one color into each soap cavity, filling them to within ¼ inch of the brim.

You will have three cubes of each color.

FINAL STEPS

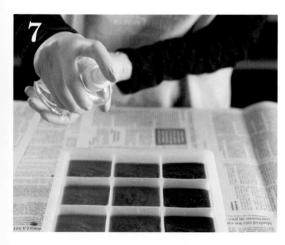

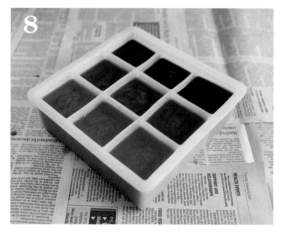

7. Spritz the mold with 99% rubbing alcohol, then cover it and force gel phase by placing it on a heating pad on medium heat for 30 minutes.

Turn off the heating pad, but leave the mold on it. Allow it to set for at least 48 hours before attempting to unmold.

8. If the soaps do not release easily from the mold, place the entire mold in the freezer for 4 hours, then try again.

Once unmolded, allow the bars to cure in a well-ventilated area for 4 to 6 weeks, turning them every few days to ensure that they cure evenly.

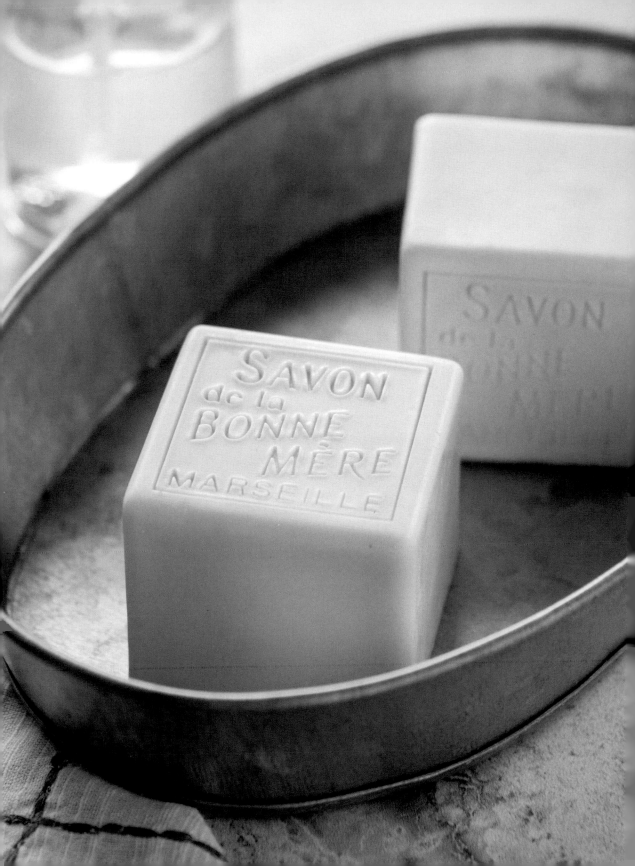

100% Castile-Brine

STAMPED CUBE

Makes 9 bars

Castile soap, a combination of pure olive oil, lye, and water, is one of the most gentle and purest forms of soap. It is not super bubbly like some recipes but has more of a slippery, low, easy lather. Castile soap improves immensely as it ages, similar to wine, and is generally considered to be at its prime after 10 months to a year. Sea salt, which has been used for hundreds of years to help improve skin conditions, helps create a harder bar.

Savon de Marseille soaps are made in France from a combination of olive oil, seawater, and lye, and this recipe is not too far from what has been tried and true for hundreds of years. The final touch of a Savon de Marseille stamp gives a traditional look.

Mold and Special Tools

- » 9-bar silicone cube
- » Savon soap stamp
- » Rubber mallet
- » Heating pad

Lye-Water Amounts

- 1 tablespoon sea salt
- 10.9 ounces distilled water
- 4.2 ounces lye (5% superfat)

Oil Amounts

- 33 ounces olive oil pure (100%)

Essential Oil Blend

- 1 ounce orange 10x essential oil
- 0.5 ounce black pepper essential oil

Safe Soaping!

Wear proper safety gear the whole time.

Work in a well-ventilated space.

No distractions (keep kids and pets away).

MAKE THE SOAP MIXTURE

1. Add the sea salt to the distilled water and stir until dissolved.

2. Add the lye to the water (never the other way around) and stir gently. Set the mixture aside to cool until it becomes clear.

3. In a bowl large enough to hold all the oil and the lye-water solution, measure out the olive oil pure.

4. When the lye-water is below 135°F (57°C), add it to the oil, pouring it over a spatula or the shaft of the stick blender to minimize air bubbles. Tap the stick blender a couple of times against the bottom of the bowl to release any air that may be trapped in the blades. *Do not turn on the stick blender until it is fully immersed.* Stick-blend for 1 minute, or until thin trace is achieved.

MIX AND POUR

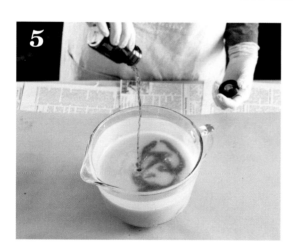

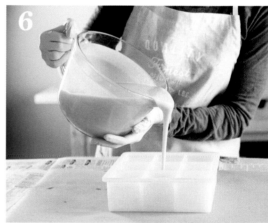

5. Slowly add the essential oil blend, and whisk until combined.

6. Pour the batter into the mold, filling each cavity approximately three-quarters of the way full.

FINAL STEPS

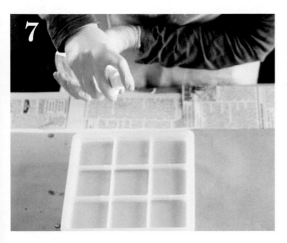

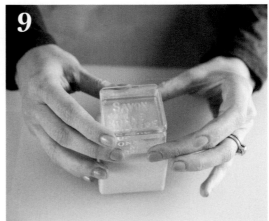

7. Spritz the top of the soaps with 99% rubbing alcohol to help prevent soda ash. Allow the soaps to sit for at least 48 to 72 hours before attempting to unmold.

8. While the salt will help this soap to set up, it may be stickier than other recipes for a few days. If you are having a hard time removing the soaps, place the entire mold in the freezer for about 4 hours, then unmold them.

9. After the soaps have been unmolded (and thawed if they were frozen), carefully line up the stamp on a cube of soap. Using a rubber mallet, firmly tap the stamp into the soap. It only needs to go in about 1/16 inch (1mm) to make a good impression. Repeat for each soap.

10. Allow the soaps to cure in a well-ventilated area for another 3 to 5 weeks before using, turning them every few days to ensure that they cure evenly.

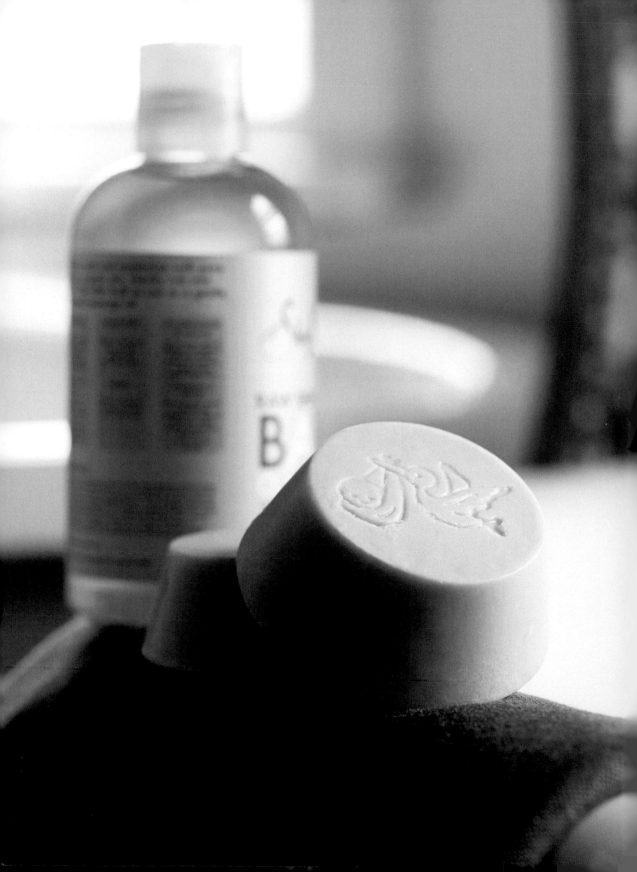

Oatmeal Soap

FOR BABIES

Makes 6 bars

Using olive oil infused with soothing chamomile, this unscented, uncolored oatmeal bar is gentle enough to cleanse and moisturize even infant skin. Chamomile is said to have calming, relaxing properties, perfect for baby's bath time. This adorable stork stamp is the perfect touch for finishing the soap for gifting or selling.

Mold and Special Tools

- » Silicone cupcake mold
- » Stamp
- » Rubber Mallet

Lye-Water Amounts

- 1.9 ounces lye (5% superfat)
- 4.3 ounces distilled water
- 1 teaspoon sodium lactate* (optional)

Oil Amounts

- 13.8 ounces chamomile-infused** olive oil pomace (92%)
- 0.8 ounce shea butter (5%)
- 0.5 ounce castor oil (3%)

Additive Amounts

- 2 teaspoons bentonite clay dispersed into 4 tablespoons distilled water
- 2 tablespoons colloidal oatmeal

This soap releases much more easily with the addition of sodium lactate.

**See instructions on next page.*

Safe Soaping!

Wear proper safety gear the whole time.

Work in a well-ventilated space.

No distractions (keep kids and pets away).

MAKE THE CHAMOMILE OIL INFUSION

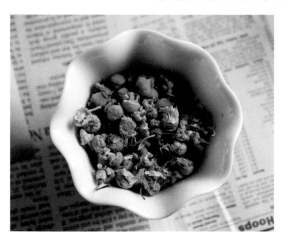 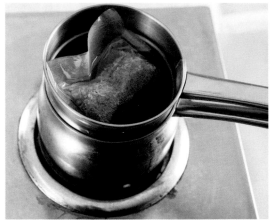

Place 2 tablespoons Egyptian chamomile into a small sealable teabag. Submerge the bag in 14.5 ounces olive oil pomace. (The amount of olive oil infused with the chamomile is larger than the recipe requires, to account for some oil that will be lost in the teabag.) Steep the oil with the teabag in a double boiler over medium heat for 2 hours before using.

MAKE THE SOAP MIXTURE

1. Add the lye to the water (never the other way around) and stir gently until all of the lye is dissolved. If using sodium lactate, add it to the lye-water and stir to combine. Set the mixture aside to cool until it becomes clear.

2. In a bowl large enough to hold all the oils and the lye-water solution, measure out the chamomile-infused olive oil. In a separate container, measure out the shea butter and castor oil and melt them together in a microwave. Be sure to heat these in 15-second bursts so as not to overheat the shea butter, stirring gently between each burst. Once the shea butter is completely melted into the castor oil, combine with the chamomile-infused olive oil in the large container.

3. When the oils and the lye-water are both below 120°F (49°C), add the lye-water to the oils, pouring it over a spatula or the shaft of the stick blender to minimize air bubbles. Tap the stick blender a couple of times against the bottom of the bowl to release any air that may be trapped in the blades. *Do not turn on the stick blender until it is fully immersed.* Stick-blend for 40 seconds, or until thin trace is achieved.

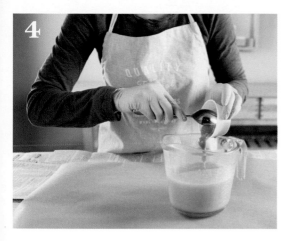

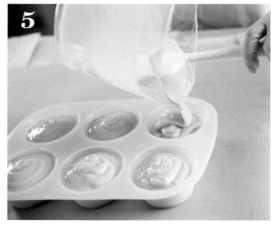

4. Add the colloidal oatmeal and all of the clay mixture. Try to trap the additives under the stick blender, and stick-blend for 15 seconds until fully blended.

5. Pour the batter into the mold, filling each cavity. Because this recipe has so much olive oil in it, it will be sticky for a few days. Spritz the top of the soaps with 99% rubbing alcohol to help prevent soda ash.

FINAL STEPS

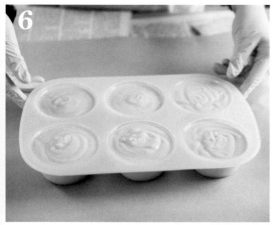

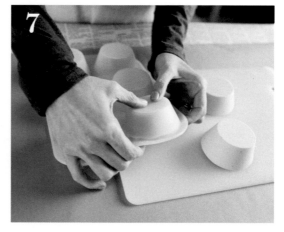

6. Allow the soaps to set for at least 3 days before attempting to unmold. If you are having a hard time removing the soaps, you can place the entire mold in the freezer for about 4 hours, and then try again.

7. After the soaps have been unmolded (and thawed if they were frozen), carefully line up the stamp on a bar of soap. Using a rubber mallet, firmly tap the stamp into the soap. It only needs to go in about 1/16 inch (1mm) to make a good impression. Repeat for each soap.

8. Allow the soaps to cure in a well-ventilated area for another 4 to 6 weeks, turning them every few days to ensure that they cure evenly.

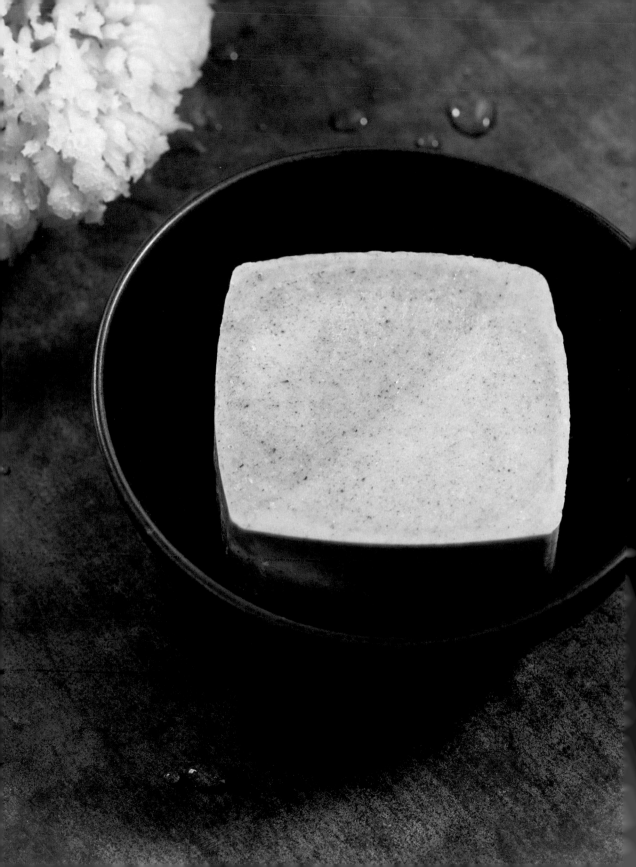

Nettle & Yarrow

UPCYCLE

Approximately 8 bars

Once you start looking for them, soap molds are everywhere, even in your recycling bin! For this recipe, we cut the top off of a milk carton to take advantage of the waxed cardboard, which acts as a pre-lined soap mold. With the addition of a simple piece of cardstock or cardboard for a divider, the mold is ready to use.

Mold

- » 1-quart cardboard milk carton (or similar waxed container)
- » 1 piece of cardboard cut to fit exactly in the diagonal of the milk carton (should be 3 3/4 inches)

Lye-Water Amounts

- 3.2 ounces lye (5% superfat)
- 7.9 ounces distilled water
- 2 teaspoons sodium lactate (optional)

Oil Amounts

- 1.2 ounces apricot kernel oil (5%)
- 0.7 ounce castor oil (3%)
- 9.4 ounces olive oil pomace (39%)
- 6 ounces rice bran oil (25%)
- 0.5 ounce shea oil (2%)
- 5.8 ounces coconut oil (24%)
- 0.5 ounce white beeswax (2%)

Colorant and Additive Amounts

- 1 teaspoon titanium dioxide dispersed into 1 tablespoon apricot kernel oil
- 2 teaspoons dried, ground nettle dispersed into 1 table-spoon apricot kernel oil
- 2 teaspoons dried yarrow pow-der dispersed into 1 table-spoon apricot kernel oil

Essential Oil Blend

- 0.2 ounce clary sage essential oil
- 0.3 ounce chamomile essential oil
- 0.5 ounce litsea cubeba essential oil

Safe Soaping!

Wear proper safety gear the whole time.

Work in a well-ventilated space.

No distractions (keep kids and pets away).

MAKE THE SOAP MIXTURE

1. Add the lye to the water (never the other way around) and stir gently until all of the lye is dissolved. If using sodium lactate, add it to the lye-water and stir to combine. Set the mixture aside to cool until it becomes clear.

2. In a bowl large enough to hold all the oils and the lye-water solution, measure out the apricot kernel oil, castor oil, olive oil pomace, rice bran oil, and shea oil. In a separate container, measure out the coconut oil and white beeswax and melt them together. Add them slowly to the liquid oils, stirring the whole time. If the beeswax and coconut oil begin to harden when added to the liquid oils, microwave them all together in 20-second bursts until the oils are all liquid.

3. When both the oils and the lye-water are between 125° and 145°F (52–63°C), add the lye-water to the oils, pouring it over a spatula or the shaft of the stick blender to minimize air bubbles. Tap the stick blender a couple of times against the bottom of the bowl to release any air that may be trapped in the blades. *Do not turn on the stick blender until it is fully immersed.* Stick-blend for 10 seconds, or until very light trace is achieved.

MIX AND POUR

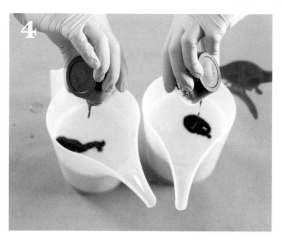

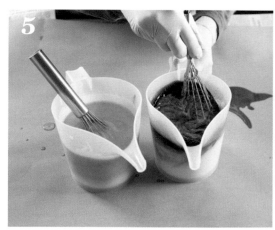

4. Add 2 teaspoons of the titanium dioxide dispersion, and whisk to combine. Split the batch equally into two containers and add the following to each container.

  » Container A: All of the nettle dispersion, and half of the essential oil
  » Container B: All of the yarrow dispersion, and half of the essential oil

5. Whisk both containers until the essential oil and additives are completely combined.

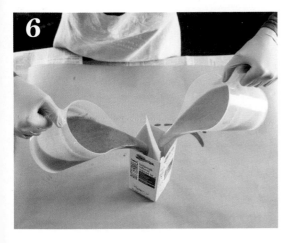

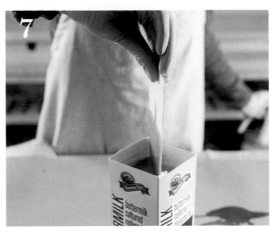

6. Simultaneously pour both of the soaps into the milk carton, one on each side of the divider.

7. Remove the divider immediately after pouring by pulling it straight up and out of the soap.

FINAL STEPS

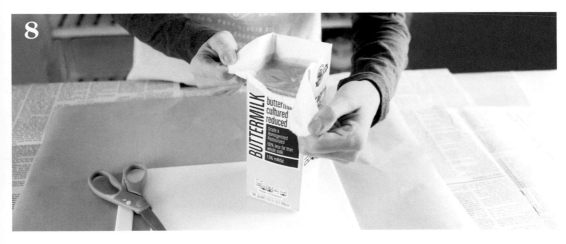

8. Gently tap the soap on the table to release any bubbles. Immediately place the entire mold into the freezer for 4 to 6 hours. After removing the soap from the freezer, let it set up for another 48 to 72 hours before unmolding.

9. To unmold, make a small cut in the upper edge of the cardboard container. From the cut, begin to tear the cardboard in a spiral pattern until it all comes free of the soap. If the cardboard is not releasing from the soap, put it back in the freezer for about 2 hours and try again.

10. Cut the soap into 1-inch thick bars. Allow the bars to cure in a well-ventilated area for 4 to 6 weeks, turning them every few days to ensure that they cure evenly.

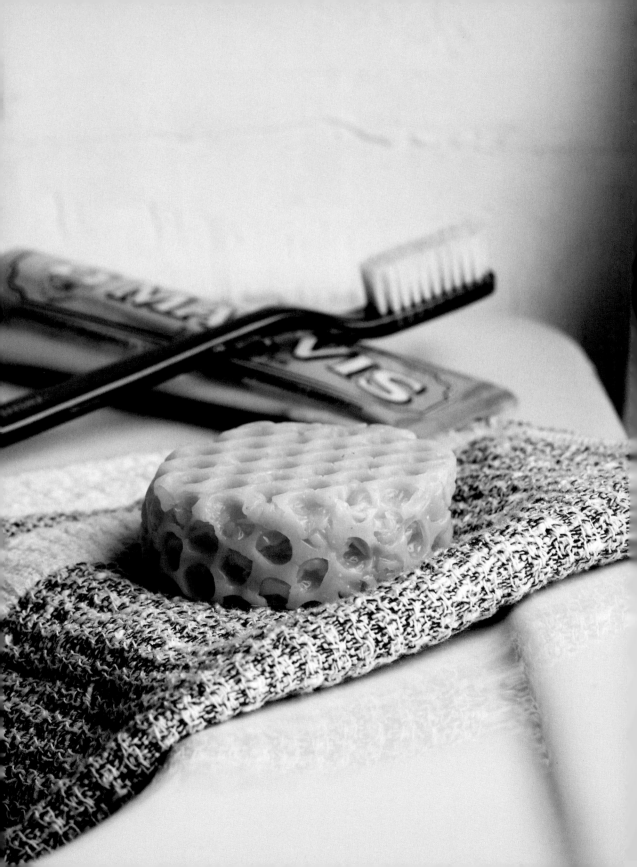

Buttermilk Honeycombs

Makes 12 bars

This adorable honeycomb soap contains a trifecta of skin goodness. Buttermilk is used around the world as a skin treatment. It is rich in lactic acid, and some say it can reduce the appearance of pores. Honey and silk combine to make a silky-smooth lather and leave skin glowing. Putting the mold in the freezer immediately after pouring prevents gel phase. If the sugars in the honey and the buttermilk scorch, it not only smells bad but will discolor the final product.

Mold and Special Tools

» 12-bar round silicone mold
» 1 (2-foot by 2-foot) sheet of small bubble wrap
» 3-inch round cookie cutter or other template
» Cutting board
» Powder sifter

Lye-Water Amounts

3.4 ounces lye (5% superfat)
4.1 ounces distilled water
1 pinch tussah silk fibers
2 teaspoons sodium lactate (optional)

Oil Amounts

10 ounces olive oil pomace (40%)
1.3 ounces avocado oil (5%)
5 ounces canola oil (20%)
2.5 ounces sunflower oil (10%)
6.3 ounces coconut oil (25%)

Additive Amounts

3 tablespoons honey
4.1 ounces buttermilk warmed to about 85°F (29°C)

Essential Oil Blend

0.5 ounce Karma essential oil blend
1 ounce orange 10x essential oil

Safe Soaping!

Wear proper safety gear the whole time.

Work in a well-ventilated space.

No distractions (keep kids and pets away).

PREPARE THE MOLDS

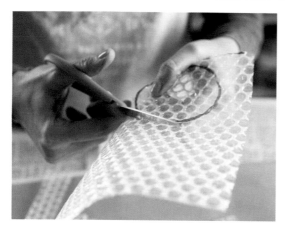

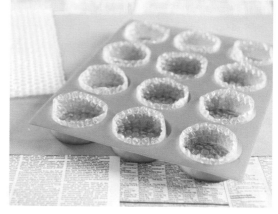

Trace the outline of a circle about 3 inches in diameter the back of the bubble wrap. Cut out the circle and use it as a template to trace and cut 11 more circles. Next, cut 12 strips, each 1½ inches wide and 9¼ inches long.

Place the round pieces in the bottom of each cavity, bumpy side up. Wrap one strip around the outside of each cavity, with the bumpy side to the middle. Place the entire mold on top of a cutting board so it is easy to transport once the soap is made.

MAKE THE SOAP MIXTURE

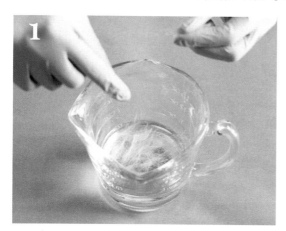

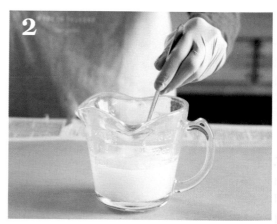

1. Measure out the water. Take a small pinch of tussah silk and pull it into individual strands. Spread the silk over the surface of the water (it will float). Add the lye to the water (never the other way around), directly over the silk fibers. The heat is an essential component to melting the silk fibers.

2. Stir gently until all of the lye and most of the fibers dissolve. If using sodium lactate, add it to the lye-water and stir to combine. Set the mixture aside to cool until it becomes clear. It is normal to have very small strands of silk floating in the lye-water.

3. In a bowl large enough to hold all the oils and the lye-water solution, measure out the olive oil pomace, avocado oil, canola oil, and sunflower oil. Place the coconut oil in the microwave in its original container, and heat until clear and liquid. Once it is completely melted, combine with the other oils.

4. When the oils and the lye-water are both below 110°F (43°C), pour the lye-water into the oils through the powder sifter to catch any undissolved silk fibers. Tap the stick blender a couple of times against the bottom of the bowl to release any air that may be trapped in the blades. *Do not turn on the stick blender until it is fully immersed.* Stick-blend to a thin trace, about 60 seconds.

MIX AND POUR

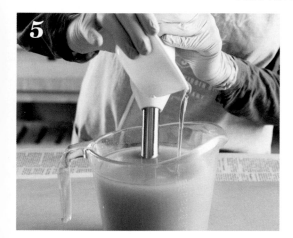

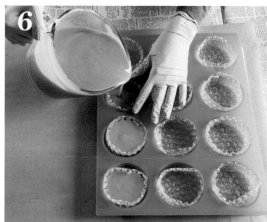

5. Add the honey, and stick-blend for 15 seconds to incorporate. Slowly pour in the slightly warmed buttermilk, then the essential oils, and whisk them into the soap until completely combined.

6. Pour the soap to fill each cavity, being careful not to disrupt the bubble wrap. Once all of the cavities are filled, gently lift the cutting board with the mold, and tamp it on the counter to release any bubbles.

FINAL STEPS

7. Immediately put the entire mold on the cutting board into the freezer for about 4 hours. Remove, and allow the soap to set at room temperature for at least 48 hours before unmolding.

8. To remove the bubble wrap from the surface of the bars, gently grasp one corner of the plastic, and pull back first the rectangular edge, then the round bottom. Place the soaps on a drying rack for 4 to 6 weeks before using, turning them every few days to ensure that they cure evenly.

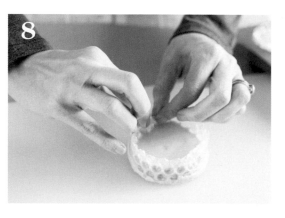

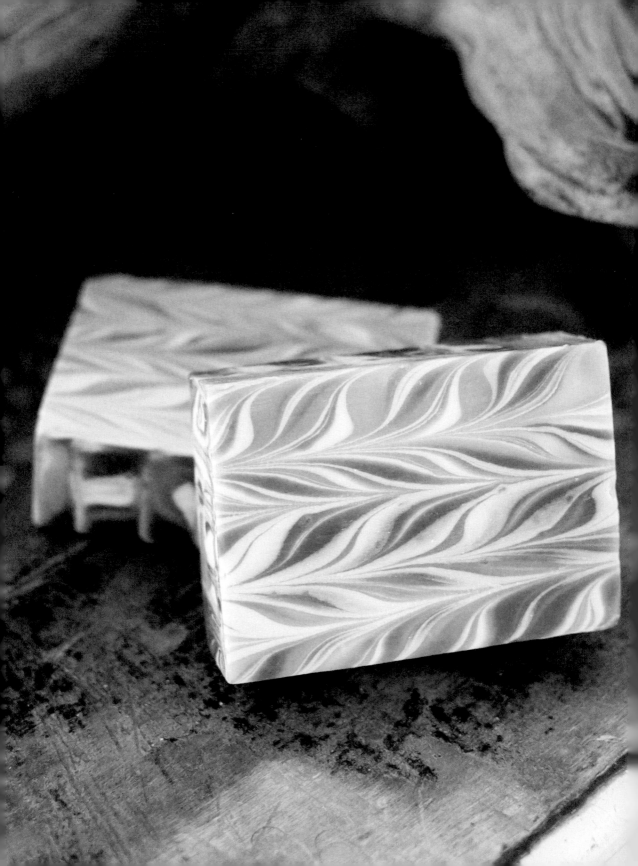

Lemon Linear

SWIRLS

Makes 18 bars

In addition to containing huge amounts of vitamin C and antioxidants, lemons are known for their deodorizing properties. While the saponification process may inhibit the deodorizing effect, the lemon zest in this soap provides a hint of exfoliation plus a burst of beautiful natural color. The cocoa powder creates a beautiful, rich brown color after going through a gel phase (see What Is Gel Phase?, page 32), so give the mold plenty of insulation to really make the colors pop.

Mold and Special Tools

» 18-bar birchwood mold with silicone liner

» Chopstick or similarly sized swirling tool

Lye-Water Amounts

7.5 ounces lye (5% superfat)

14.1 ounces distilled water

1½ tablespoons sodium lactate (optional)

Oil Amounts

9.2 ounces palm oil (17%)

9.2 ounces coconut oil (17%)

1.2 ounces deodorized cocoa butter (2%)

3 ounces palm kernel flakes (5%)

15.3 ounces olive oil pure (28%)

9.2 ounces rice bran oil (17%)

7.9 ounces sweet almond oil (14%)

Essential Oil Blend

2 ounces bergamot essential oil

2 ounces litsea cubeba essential oil

Colorant and Additive Amounts

1–2 large lemons, zest and juice (seeds strained out; 4 ounces total)

1 teaspoon annatto seeds infused in 1 ounce of sweet almond oil*

2 teaspoons Dutch-process cocoa powder dispersed into 2 tablespoons sweet almond oil

2 teaspoons titanium dioxide dispersed into 2 tablespoons sweet almond oil

See pages 48–49 for how to make infused oils.

Safe Soaping!

Wear proper safety gear the whole time.

Work in a well-ventilated space.

No distractions (keep kids and pets away).

MAKE THE SOAP MIXTURE

1. Add the lye to the water (never the other way around) and stir gently until all of the lye is dissolved. If using sodium lactate, add it to the lye-water and stir to combine. Set the mixture aside to cool until it becomes clear.

2. Melt the palm oil in its original container, mix it thoroughly, and measure into a bowl large enough to hold all of the oils and the lye-water with room for mixing. Melt and measure the coconut oil and add it to the bowl. Add the cocoa butter and palm kernel flakes to the hot oils, and stir until melted. If needed, heat the oils further until the butter and flakes are melted.

Add the olive oil pure, rice bran oil, and sweet almond oil.

3. When both the oils and the lye-water are between 110° and 120°F (43–49°C), add the lye-water to the oils, pouring it over a spatula or the shaft of the stick blender to minimize air bubbles. Tap the stick blender a couple of times against the bottom of the bowl to release any air that may be trapped in the blades. *Do not turn on the stick blender until it is fully immersed.* Stick-blend for 20 seconds, or until thin trace is achieved.

MIX IN THE ADDITIVES

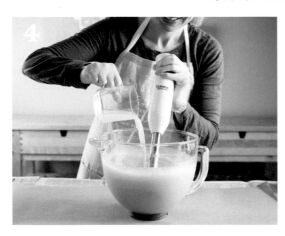

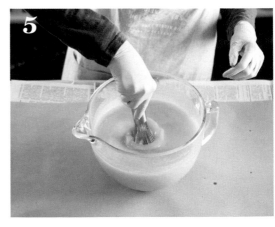

4. Add the lemon juice and zest to the batter. Stick-blend for 10 seconds. The batter will turn a lovely orange/yellow.

5. Add the essential oil blend, and whisk to combine.

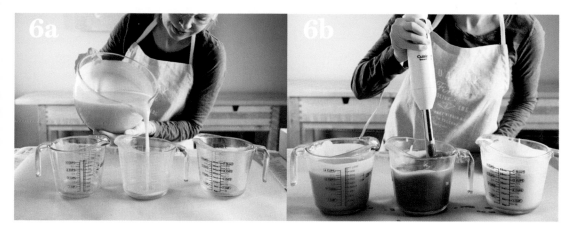

6. Divide the soap into three equal parts and add the colorants as follows.

» Container A: annatto infusion
» Container B: all of the Dutch-process cocoa powder dispersion
» Container C: all of the titanium dioxide dispersion

Stick-blend each container about 2 seconds, just long enough to incorporate the colors.

POUR AND SWIRL

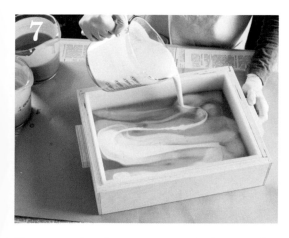

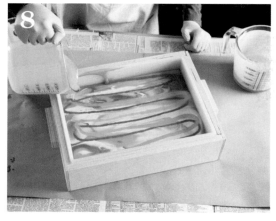

7. Pour random S-curves across the bottom of the mold, using a different color for each one and varying the amount of soap used for each pour. Do this with approximately half of each color.

8. With the remaining batter, pour thin lines of soap lengthwise across the mold so the entire surface is covered.

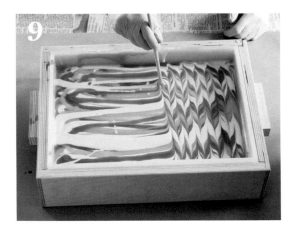

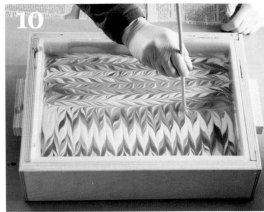

9. With the mold positioned lengthwise, insert a chopstick in the top left corner until it reaches the bottom of the mold. Drag the chopstick perpendicular to the lines of the soap, making S-curves until it reaches the other edge of the mold.

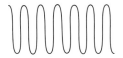

10. Insert the chopstick in the far left corner again, all the way to the bottom of the mold. This time, drag the chopstick lengthwise along the wall of the mold, moving in the same direction as the original stripes of soap. Create S-curves in this manner across the entire soap.

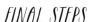

FINAL STEPS

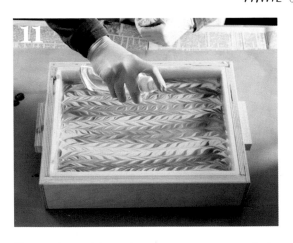

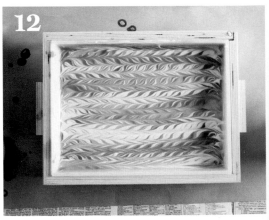

11. Tap the mold to release any remaining air bubbles. Spritz the top of the soap with 99% rubbing alcohol. Cover the mold, and carefully drape a towel over it. This soap should go through gel phase to achieve the brightest color. Allow it to set for 48 hours before attempting to unmold.

12. Cut the soap into bars using a sharp knife. Allow the bars to cure in a well-ventilated area for 4 to 6 weeks before using, turning them every few days to ensure that they cure evenly.

Banana Cream Pie
LAYERED BARS

Approximately 12 bars

With bananas and heavy cream, this soap is as good as the dessert but without the calories! Temperature plays a big role here, because the natural sugars in the bananas and the whipping cream cause the main soap batter to heat up, which can then "melt" the whipped topping. Keep the main batter temperatures as low as possible, and move this soap to the freezer quickly after finishing the topping to avoid partial gel phase or overheating (see What Is Gel Phase?, page 32).

STAGE 1
PREPARE THE WHIPPED TOPPING

Lye-Water Amounts
- 1.6 ounces lye (2% superfat)
- 3.6 ounces distilled water

Oil Amounts
- 3.3 ounces palm oil (30%)
- 2.8 ounces coconut oil (25%)
- 1.7 ounces mango butter (15%)
- 1.1 ounces cocoa butter (10%)
- 1.1 ounces olive oil pomace (10%)
- 1.1 ounces palm kernel flakes (10%)

Colorant and Additive Amounts
- 1 teaspoon titanium dioxide dispersed into 1 tablespoon sweet almond oil

Essential Oil Blend
- 0.5 ounce balsam Peru essential oil

Safe Soaping!

Wear proper safety gear the whole time.

Work in a well-ventilated space.

No distractions (keep kids and pets away).

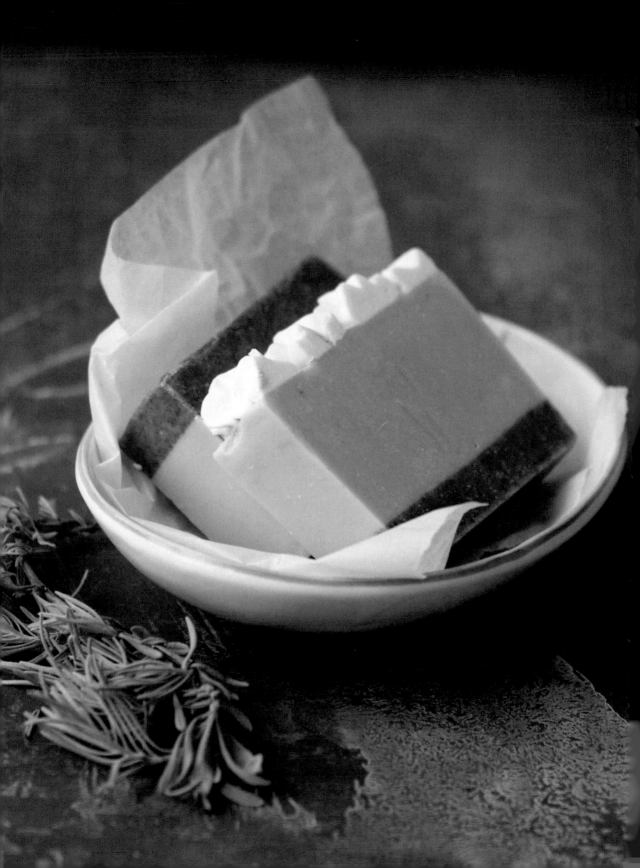

MAKE THE SOAP MIXTURE

1. Add the lye to the water (never the other way around) and stir gently until all of the lye is dissolved. Place the cup in a cool-water bath in a safe place.

2. Melt the palm oil in its original container, mix it thoroughly, and measure into a bowl that will hold at least 48 ounces to ensure room for mixing.

3. Melt and measure the coconut oil and add it to the bowl. Add the mango butter, cocoa butter, and palm kernel flakes to the hot oils and stir until melted. If needed, heat the oils further until the butter and flakes are melted. Add the olive oil pomace, and stir to combine.

4. Place the bowl in an ice-water bath and set it aside.

STAGE 2

MAKE THE BASE SOAP

Mold and Special Tools

» 10-inch silicone loaf mold
» Electric hand mixer
» Disposable frosting bag
» 1M frosting tip

Lye-Water Amounts

4.8 ounces lye (5% superfat)
7.3 ounces distilled water
1 tablespoon sodium lactate (optional)

Oil Amounts

6.3 ounces palm oil (18%)
8.8 ounces coconut oil (25%)
1.8 ounces shea butter (5%)
1.8 ounces apricot kernel oil (5%)
12.3 ounces olive oil pure (35%)
4.2 ounces rice bran oil (12%)

Colorant and Additive Amounts

1.2 ounces banana, 1.5 ounces whipping cream, and 1.5 ounces water, pureed in a blender until smooth

1 1/2 tablespoons ground walnut shells

1 teaspoon yellow oxide dispersed into 1 tablespoon sweet almond oil

1 teaspoon titanium dioxide dispersed into 1 tablespoon sweet almond oil

Essential Oil Blend

0.2 ounce cinnamon essential oil
1.6 ounces balsam Peru essential oil

MAKE THE SOAP MIXTURE

1. Add the lye to the water (never the other way around) and stir gently until all of the lye is dissolved. If using sodium lactate, add it to the lye-water and stir to combine. Set the mixture aside to cool until it becomes clear.

2. Melt the palm oil in its original container, mix it thoroughly, and measure into a bowl large enough to hold all of the oils and the lye-water with room for mixing. Melt and measure the coconut oil and add it to the bowl. Add the shea butter to the hot oils and stir until melted. If needed, heat the oils further until the shea butter is fully melted. Add the apricot kernel, olive oil pure, and rice bran oil.

3. When both the oils and lye-water are between 80° and 90°F (27–32°C), add the lye-water to the oils, pouring it over a spatula or the shaft of the stick blender to minimize air bubbles. Tap the stick blender a couple of times against the bottom of the bowl to release any air that may be trapped in the blades. *Do not turn on the stick blender until it is fully immersed.* Stick-blend for 30 seconds, or until thin trace is achieved.

MIX AND POUR

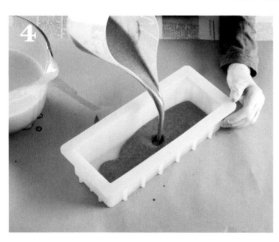 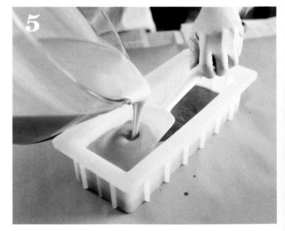

4. Add the banana puree to the soap batter. Stick-blend for another 15 seconds. Pour 1 ½ cups (350ml) of the soap batter into an easy-pour container. Add the walnut shells and one-fourth of the essential oil blend, and stick-blend together for 15 seconds. Pour the batter into the mold, and tamp the mold on the table.

5. To the main batch, whisk in 2 teaspoons yellow dispersion, 2 tablespoons white dispersion, and the rest of the essential oil blend. Stick-blend for 5 seconds. Pour the batter over a spatula onto the first layer, slowly and gently to avoid breaking through the layer.

Gently tamp the mold on the table to bring any air bubbles to the surface. Set the soap aside.

FINISH THE WHIPPED TOPPING

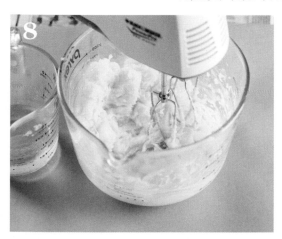

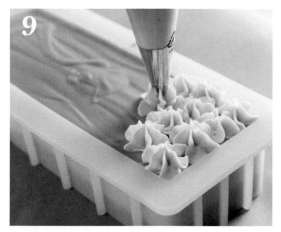

6. Remove the lye solution and the oils for the whipped topping from their cold-water baths. You want the oils to be a bit firm, but not solid. Using a hand mixer, whip the oils on medium for 20 seconds, or until a smooth consistency is achieved. Slowly add the cool lye-water into the oils.

7. Taking care not to splash, stick-blend for 30 seconds, then add the balsam Peru essential oil and the titanium dioxide dispersion. Stick-blend for another 45 seconds or until very thick trace is achieved.

8. Use the hand mixer on high speed to whip the soap for 5 minutes, or until the batter forms stiff peaks.

9. Spoon the batter into a frosting bag with the 1M tip attached. Pipe small peaks along the soap, about ½ inch high. Four peaks fit nicely side by side along the short side of the mold. Repeat this across the entire surface of the soap.

FINAL STEPS

10. Place the entire soap in the freezer for 24 hours to avoid overheating from the sugars in the banana. After removing the soap from the freezer, allow the soap to sit at room temperature for another 24 hours before unmolding. Because of the temperature changes, the soap will become very wet with condensation, but it will dry off again after a few hours.

11. Unmold the soap, and cut into bars. Allow the soap to cure in a well-ventilated area for 4 to 6 weeks before using, turning them every few days to ensure that they cure evenly.

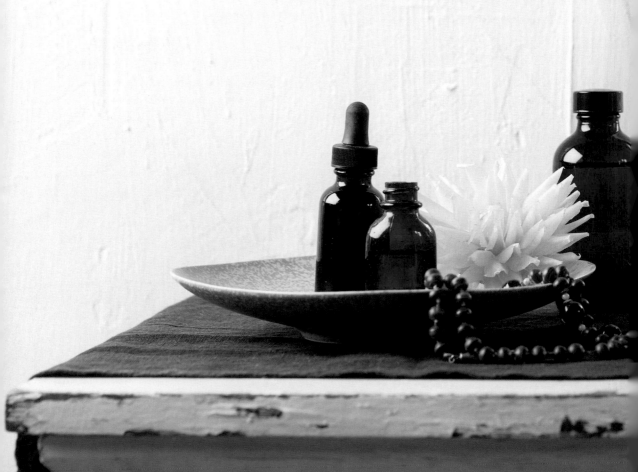

CHAPTER 9

Pure Beauty

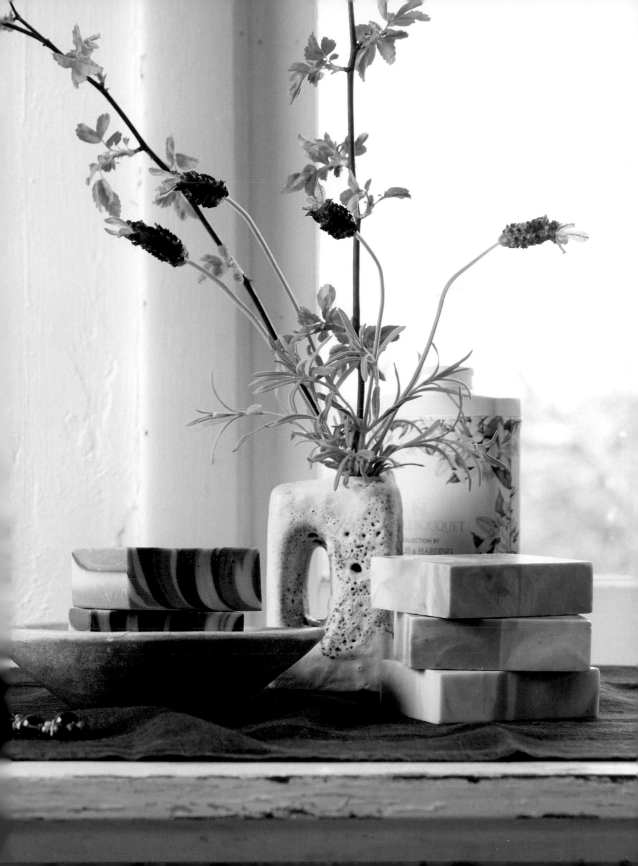

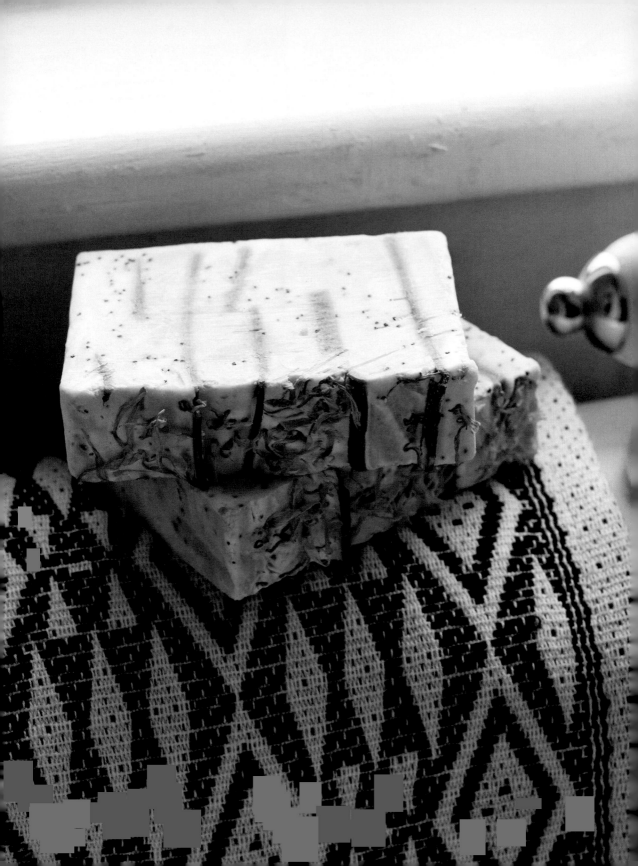

Annatto-Yarrow

WITH EMBEDS

Approximately 12 bars

This recipe uses a number of herbs and several different techniques, but it is not complicated to make. It calls for an annatto oil infusion, a yarrow lye-water infusion, and embeds that need to be made ahead of time.

Annatto is used in many foods and cosmetics for the beautiful pop of orange it provides. An ancient remedy used as a wound healer, yarrow has been found in burial sites as old as 60,000 BCE. Today, many people use it to improve circulation and soothe skin irritation, but it should be avoided during pregnancy.

STAGE 1

MAKE THE EMBEDS

Mold and Special Tools

» 10-inch silicone loaf mold
» Cheese slicer

Lye-Water Amounts

1 ounce lye (5% superfat)
2.3 ounces distilled water
½ teaspoon sodium lactate (optional)

Oil Amounts

1.8 ounces palm oil (25%)
1.8 ounces coconut oil (25%)
0.5 ounce mango butter (7%)
3 ounces olive oil pomace (43%)

Colorant and Additive Amounts

1 tablespoon spirulina powder
1 teaspoon yarrow powder

Essential Oil

0.3 ounce bergamot essential oil

Note: This beautiful design requires that the embeds cure for 48 hours before using them in the base soap, so plan ahead.

Safe Soaping!

Wear proper safety gear the whole time.

Work in a well-ventilated space.

No distractions (keep kids and pets away).

MAKE THE SOAP MIXTURE

1. Add the lye to the water (never the other way around) and stir gently until all of the lye is dissolved. If using sodium lactate, add it to the lye-water and stir to combine. Set aside until clear.

2. Add the spirulina and yarrow powder directly to the hot lye-water, and stir until there are no more clumps.

Melt the palm oil in its original container, mix it thoroughly, and measure into a bowl large enough to hold all of the oils and the lye-water with room for mixing. Melt and measure the coconut oil and add it to the bowl. Add mango butter to the hot oils, and stir until melted. If needed, microwave in 10-second bursts until completely melted. Add the olive oil pomace to the hot oils.

3. When the oils and the lye-water are between 110° and 120°F (43–49°C), add the lye-water to the oils, pouring it over a spatula or the shaft of the stick blender to minimize air bubbles. Tap the stick blender a couple of times against the bottom of the bowl to release any air that may be trapped in the blades. *Do not turn on the stick blender until it is fully immersed.* Stick-blend for 10 seconds, or until very thin trace is achieved.

4. Add all of the essential oil and stick-blend for 5 seconds.

5. Pour the batter into the mold; it should just be a thin layer of soap. Tap the mold to settle the soap, and let it set for 48 hours before attempting to unmold.

CUT THE EMBEDS

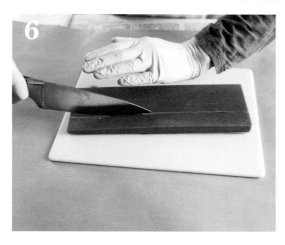

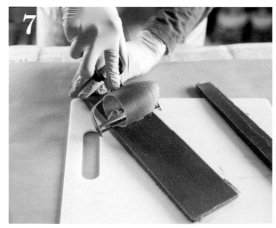

6. Once unmolded, cut the soap lengthwise to create two pieces, with one piece being twice as wide as the other (roughly one-third and two-thirds).

7. Use a cheese slicer to cut both pieces into slices of various thicknesses. Having different-sized embeds creates a unique look to each bar.

STAGE 2

STAGE 2
MAKE THE BASE SOAP

Mold and Special Tools

» 10-inch silicone loaf mold

Lye-Water Amounts

4.7 ounces lye (5% superfat)

11.2 ounces distilled water

1 tablespoon sodium lactate (optional)

Oil Amounts

6.8 ounces palm oil (20%)

8.5 ounces coconut oil (25%)

10.2 ounces olive oil pure (30%)

6.8 ounces rice bran oil (20%)

1.7 ounces chia seed oil (5%)

Essential Oil Blend

0.8 ounce bergamot essential oil

0.8 ounce rosemary essential oil

Colorant and Additive Amounts

2 tablespoons poppy seeds

1 tablespoon annatto seeds infused in 1 ounce olive oil pure*

2 heaping tablespoons calendula petals

Embed slices (made 48 hours before)

See pages 48–49 for how to make infused oils.

MAKE THE SOAP MIXTURE

1. Add the lye to the water (never the other way around) and stir gently until all of the lye is dissolved. If using sodium lactate, add it to the lye-water and stir to combine. Set the mixture aside to cool until it becomes clear.

2. Melt the palm oil in its original container, mix it thoroughly, and measure into a bowl large enough to hold all of the oils and the lye-water with room for mixing. Melt and measure the coconut oil and add it to the bowl. Add the olive oil pure, rice bran oil, and chia seed oil to the hot oils.

3. When the oils and the lye-water are between 110° and 120°F (43–49°C), add the lye-water to the oils, pouring it over a spatula or the shaft of the stick blender to minimize air bubbles. Tap the stick blender a couple of times against the bottom of the bowl to release any air that may be trapped in the blades. *Do not turn on the stick blender until it is fully immersed.* Stick-blend for 45 seconds, or until thin trace is achieved.

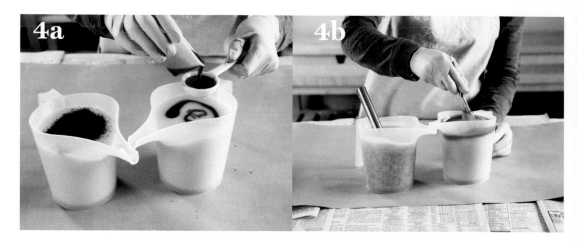

4. Add all of the essential oil to the batter and whisk to combine.

Split the batch in half, add the following to each container, then whisk to combine:
   » Container A: all the poppy seeds
   » Container B: 2 tablespoons annatto infusion

POUR THE SOAP

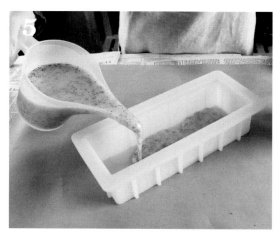

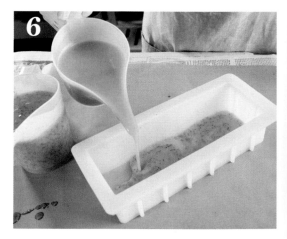

5. Beginning with the poppy seed batter, pour across the bottom of the mold in an S pattern, using only about a cup of batter.

6. Repeat this process with the yellow batter, pouring it into the poppy seed batter. Continue alternating pours of poppy seed and annatto batter until all of the batter is used.

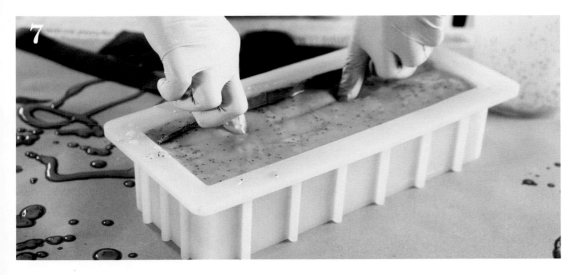

7. Insert the green embeds, pushing them into the soap like grass blades in a random fashion. Tap the mold firmly on the counter to settle the soap and release any bubbles.

FINAL STEPS

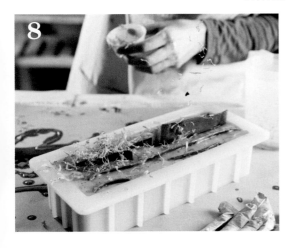

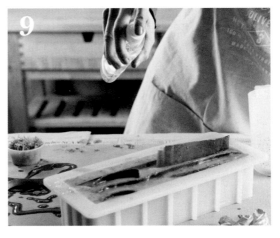

8. Finish off the soap with a sprinkling of calendula petals across the entire surface of the soap. If needed, use a spoon to gently push the petals securely into the soap.

9. Spritz with 99% rubbing alcohol to help prevent soda ash. Allow the soap to set for 2 to 3 days before attempting to unmold.

10. To cut into bars, turn the block on its side to avoid dragging petals down through the soap as you cut. Allow the bars to cure in a well-ventilated area for 4 to 6 weeks before using, turning them every few days to ensure that they cure evenly.

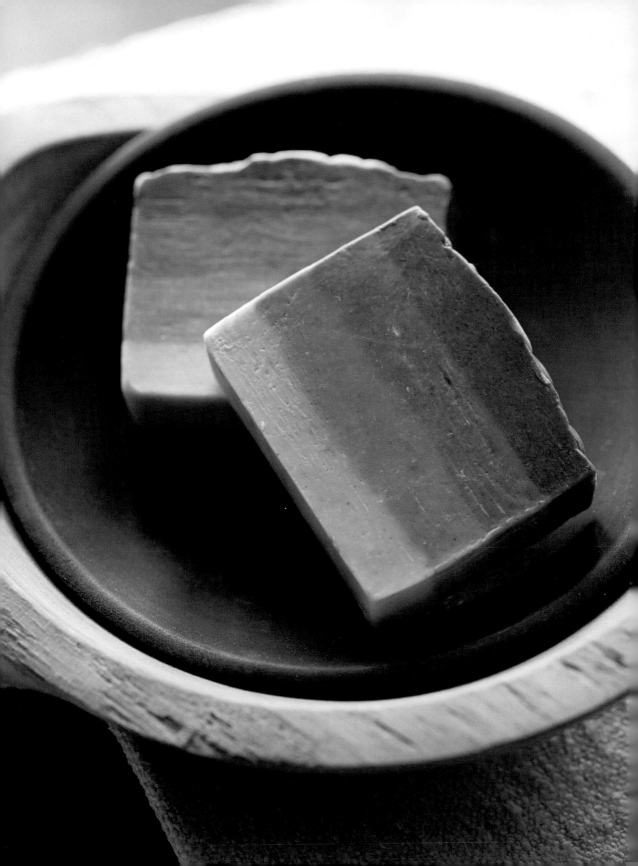

Madder Root
OMBRE BARS

Approximately 8 bars

Powdered madder root has a rich red color. It belongs in the same family as coffee and is a natural astringent. To achieve the ombre effect, pour each layer low and slow over a spatula to keep the lines nice and straight. To bring out the best color for this soap, a hot gel phase is essential. Soaping at slightly higher temperatures than in typical recipes and using good insulation will ensure a full gel (see What Is Gel Phase?, page 32).

Mold and Special Tools

- » 2-pound wooden mold with silicone liner
- » Squirt bottle
- » Chopstick or similarly sized swirling tool
- » Heating pad

Lye-Water Amounts

- 3 ounces lye (5% superfat)
- 7.3 ounces distilled water
- 2 teaspoons sodium lactate (optional)

Oil Amounts

- 5.5 ounces palm oil (25%)
- 5.5 ounces coconut oil (25%)
- 0.7 ounce cocoa butter (3%)
- 5.5 ounces olive oil pure (25%)
- 4.8 ounces rice bran oil (22%)

Additive Amounts

- 2 teaspoons titanium dioxide dispersed into 2 tablespoons olive oil pure
- 3 tablespoons of madder root dispersed into 2 ounces olive oil pure

Essential Oil Blend

- 0.5 ounce black pepper essential oil
- 0.5 ounce lemongrass essential oil

Safe Soaping!

Wear proper safety gear the whole time.

Work in a well-ventilated space.

No distractions (keep kids and pets away).

MAKE THE SOAP MIXTURE

1. Add the lye to the water (never the other way around) and stir gently until all of the lye is dissolved. If using sodium lactate, add it to the lye-water and stir to combine. Set the mixture aside to cool until it becomes clear.

2. Melt the palm oil in its original container, mix it thoroughly, and measure into a bowl large enough to hold all of the oils and the lye-water with room for mixing. Melt and measure the coconut oil and add it to the bowl. Add the cocoa butter to the hot oils. Stir until melted. If needed, heat the oils further until the cocoa butter is melted. Add the olive oil pure and rice bran oil to the other oils.

3. When both the oils and the lye-water are between 120° and 130°F (49–54°C), add the lye-water to the oils, pouring it over a spatula or the shaft of the stick blender to minimize air bubbles. Tap the stick blender a couple of times against the bottom of the bowl to release any air that may be trapped in the blades. *Do not turn on the stick blender until it is fully immersed.* Stick-blend for 30 seconds, or until very thin trace is achieved.

4. Pour about ¼ cup of batter into a squirt bottle. Set aside.

MIX AND POUR

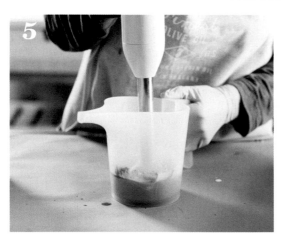

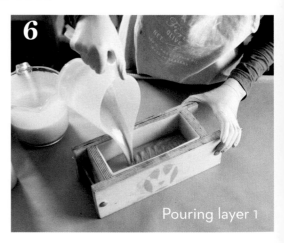

Pouring layer 1

5. For the first layer, pour about 1 cup of batter into an easy-pour container. Add to the batter:
  » 1 teaspoon of titanium dioxide dispersion
  » ¼ teaspoon madder root dispersion
  » One-fourth of the essential oil blend

Using a whisk, blend the batter until the color and essential oil are completely mixed in. Stick-blend for 5 seconds to help soap set up.

6. Gently pour the batter into the mold, and tamp the mold until the layer is flat.

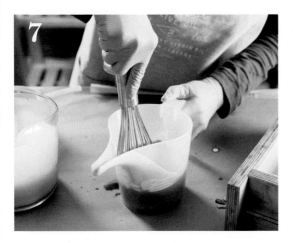

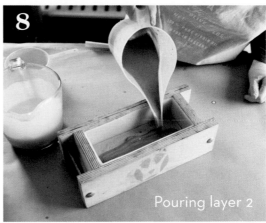

Pouring layer 2

7. For the second layer, pour 1 cup of batter into the same container and add:

> » 1 teaspoon titanium dioxide blend
> » 1½ teaspoons madder root dispersion
> » One-third of the remaining essential oil

Whisk the batter until the color and essential oil are completely dispersed. Stick-blend for 5 seconds.

8. Gently pour the batter over the first layer, pouring as low as possible and very slowly to allow the batter to spread over the first layer and cover it completely. Gently tap the mold on the table to release any air bubbles.

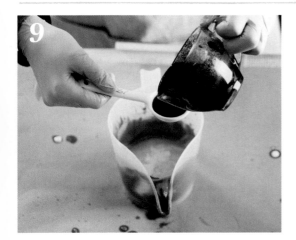

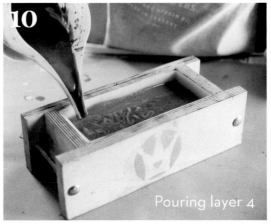

Pouring layer 4

9. For the third layer, pour 1 cup of batter into the container and add:

> » 1 teaspoon titanium dioxide blend
> » 1 tablespoon madder root dispersion
> » Half of the remaining essential oil

Whisk the batter until the color and essential oil are completely mixed in and pour the third layer as described in step 8.

10. For the final layer, pour the last of the batter into the container and add:

> » 1 teaspoon titanium dioxide blend
> » 2 tablespoons madder root dispersion
> » Remaining essential oil

Whisk the batter until the color and essential oil are completely mixed in and pour the final layer as described in step 8.

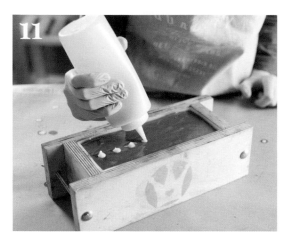

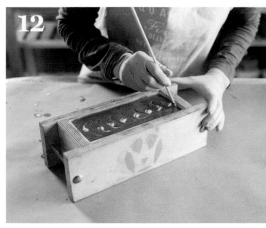

11. Gently shake the squirt bottle to loosen the soap, and squirt dots down the center of the soap, roughly ½ inch apart.

12. Insert the wide end of a chopstick about ¼ inch into the soap, starting on the edge of the mold, next to the white dots. Move the chopstick through the dots in a figure eight pattern, dragging the white through the purple soap.

FINAL STEPS

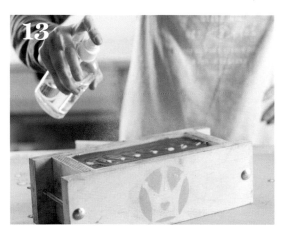

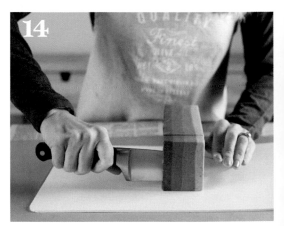

13. Spritz the soap with 99% rubbing alcohol, and place the mold on a heating pad on medium for 30 minutes, covered. Turn off the pad, but leave the soap insulated and on top of the warm pad overnight. Allow the soap to set for at least 48 hours before attempting to unmold.

14. To cut this soap, turn the loaf on its side so that the cuts run with the layers; this will keep the layers from dragging into each other. Allow the bars to cure in a well-ventilated area for 4 to 6 weeks before using, turning them every few days to ensure that they cure evenly.

Cucumber Layers

Approximately 8 bars

The simple cucumber is packed with skin-loving vitamins: C, B_1, B_2, B_3, and B_5. Some soapmakers report that cucumber accelerates trace, so double-check that the mold and all of the necessary spoons and containers are ready for action before beginning to make this soap. This recipe works with the acceleration and is designed to hold a tall peak that will not sag.

Mold and Special Tools

» 2-pound wooden loaf mold with silicone liner
» Heating pad
» Large piece of cardboard

Lye-Water Amounts

2.9 ounces lye (5% superfat)

6.1 ounces distilled water

2 teaspoons sodium lactate (optional)

Oil Amounts

17.6 ounces olive oil pure (80%)

3.3 ounces coconut oil (15%)

1.1 ounces shea butter (5%)

Colorant and Additive Amounts

1 ounce cucumber puree (2-ounce chunk of peeled cucumber, seeds included, pureed in a blender until smooth)

1 tablespoon cucumber skin, pureed until mostly smooth

1 tablespoon spirulina powder dispersed into 1 tablespoon olive oil pure

1 teaspoon titanium dioxide dispersed into 1 tablespoon olive oil pure

1 tablespoon annatto seeds infused in 1 ounce olive oil pure (see pages 48–49)

Optional Color Palette

For a more intense color, replace the spirulina powder and the annatto infusion with the following:

1 teaspoon green chrome oxide dispersed into 1 tablespoon olive oil pure

1 teaspoon yellow oxide dispersed into 1 tablespoon olive oil pure

Essential Oil Blend

0.7 ounce lavender 40/42 essential oil*

0.3 ounce patchouli essential oil

Regular lavender essential oil will work, but this variety has been specifically blended to last in cold-process soap.

Safe Soaping!

Wear proper safety gear the whole time.

Work in a well-ventilated space.

No distractions (keep kids and pets away).

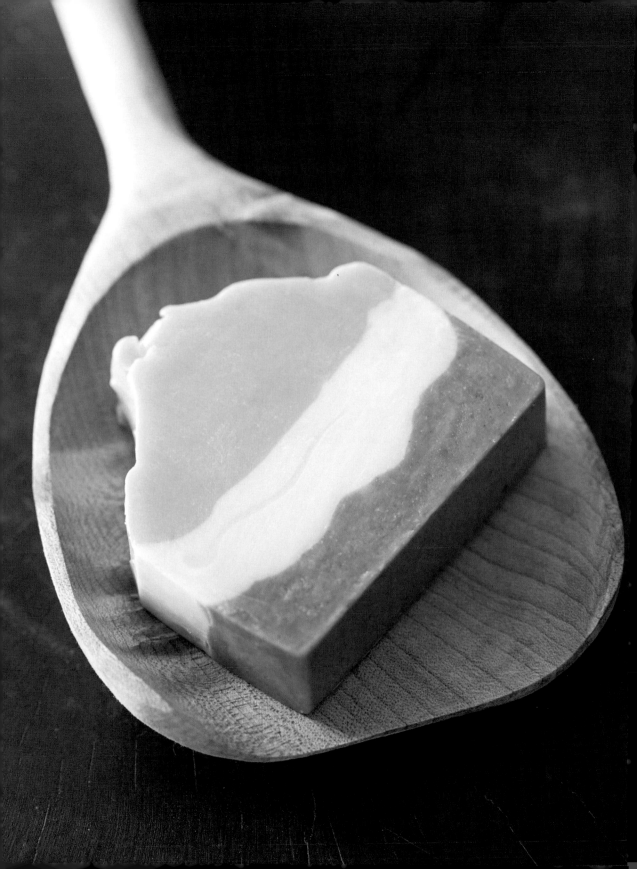

MAKE THE SOAP MIXTURE

1. Add the lye to the water (never the other way around) and stir gently until all of the lye is dissolved. Add the sodium lactate to the lye-water and stir to combine. Set the mixture aside to cool until it becomes clear.

2. In a bowl large enough to hold all the oils and the lye-water solution, measure out the olive oil pure. In a separate container, measure out and melt the coconut oil and shea butter. Once they are completely melted, combine with the other oils in the large bowl.

3. When both the oils and the lye-water have cooled to between 110° and 120°F (43–49°C), add the lye-water to the oils, pouring it over a spatula or the shaft of the stick blender to minimize air bubbles. Tap the stick blender a couple of times against the bottom of the bowl to release any air that may be trapped in the blades. *Do not turn on the stick blender until the blades are fully immersed.* Stick-blend for about 45 seconds, or until thin trace is achieved.

MIX AND POUR

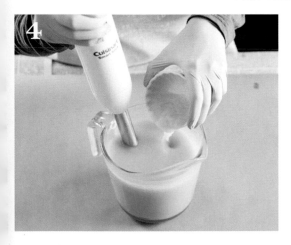

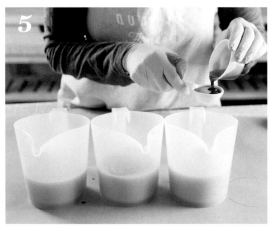

4. Add one ounce of the light green cucumber puree to the batter, and stick-blend for 5 seconds.

5. Divide the batter equally among three containers. Color the containers as follows.

>» Container A: 1 tablespoon dark green cucumber-skin puree, 1 tablespoon spirulina dispersion (or green chrome oxide dispersion)

>» Container B: 1 teaspoon titanium dioxide dispersion

>» Container C: 4 teaspoons annatto-infused oil (or yellow oxide dispersion)

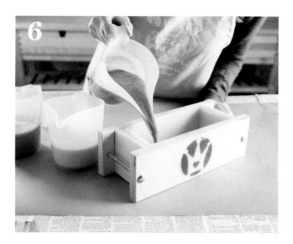

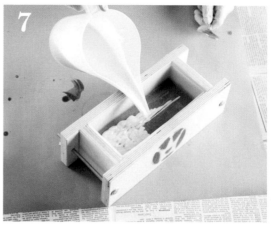

6. Pour approximately one-third of the essential oil blend into the dark green soap. Stick-blend this into the batter for 3 seconds. Pour the green soap into the lined mold.

7. Pour approximately one-third of the essential oil blend into the white soap. Whisk the essential oils into the soap. Carefully pour the white soap low and slow over the green soap, so that the second layer doesn't break through. (Pour over the back of a clean spatula if it isn't quite thick enough.)

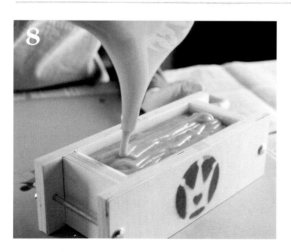

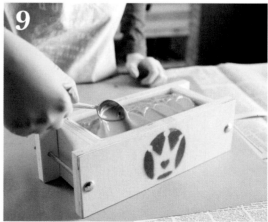

8. Repeat with the orange soap, again using a spatula if necessary to keep it from breaking into the white layer.

9. Using the back of a spoon, build texture on the top of the soap. Pull the soap from the outer edges of the mold, up toward the center into a peak. If the soap is not quite solid enough to hold its shape, wait a minute or two and try again.

FINAL STEPS

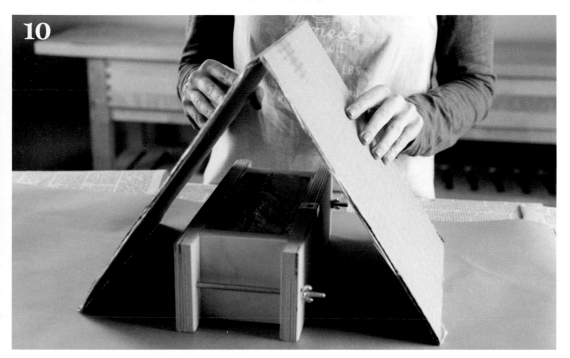

10. Set the soap on top of a heating pad (not shown here) turned on low in an out-of-the-way spot. Place a cardboard "tent" over the soap so it is not touching your creation, and carefully drape a small towel over it. Leave the heating pad on for 20 minutes, then turn it off, but don't move the soap.

11. After 48 hours, unmold the soap and cut it into bars. To cut, turn the soap on its side to avoid dragging the layers into each other. Allow the bars to cure in a cool, dark, well-ventilated area for 4 to 6 weeks before using, turning them every few days to ensure that they cure evenly.

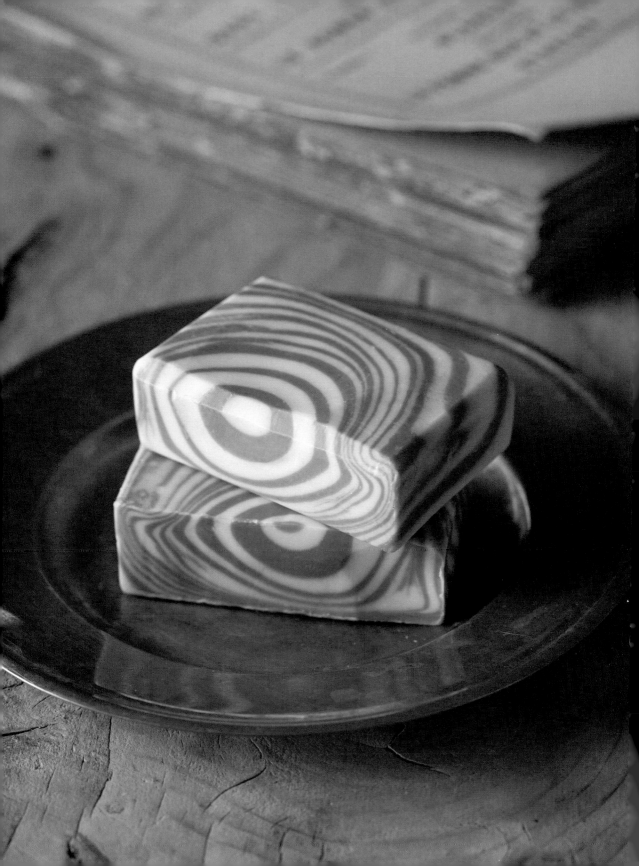

White Tea

FAUX FUNNEL POUR

Makes 9 bars

The beautiful concentric swirls of this soap are created using a technique called "faux funnel pour." A thin trace and random placement of centers for the pour combine to create the fine lines. White tea is the least processed type of tea, and it retains the highest content of catechins, powerful antioxidants that are often used in anti-aging creams. The tea is frozen to help prevent it from scorching and turning an even darker color in the soap. Keeping a neutral color palette is essential for pulling off this design with aplomb.

Mold and Special Tools

- » 9-bar birchwood mold and liner
- » 2 squirt bottles

Lye-Water Amounts

- 4.5 ounces lye (5% superfat)
- 10.8 ounces white tea made with distilled water, frozen into cubes
- 1 tablespoon sodium lactate (optional)

Oil Amounts

- 7.8 ounces coconut oil (23%)
- 2.3 ounces shea butter (7%)
- 16.5 ounces olive oil pure (50%)
- 6.6 ounces canola oil (20%)

Essential Oil Amount

- 1.5 ounces eucalyptus essential oil

Colorant Amounts

- 1 teaspoon titanium dioxide dispersed into 1 tablespoon canola oil
- 1 teaspoon green chrome oxide dispersed into 1 tablespoon canola oil

Safe Soaping!

Wear proper safety gear the whole time.

Work in a well-ventilated space.

No distractions (keep kids and pets away).

MAKE THE SOAP MIXTURE

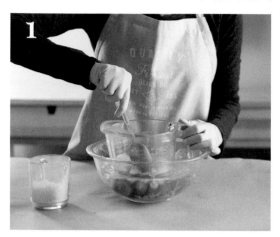

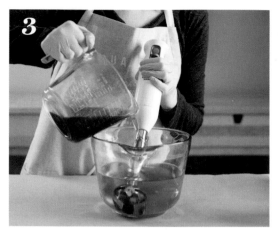

1. Place the white tea ice cubes in a heat-safe container and put the container in a cold-water bath. Slowly sprinkle approximately 1 tablespoon of lye over the tea. Carefully stir until the lye is beginning to dissolve. Add another tablespoon of lye to the mixture, and continue stirring. Repeat this process until all of the lye is dissolved. The mixture will have an odd smell and color to it, which is normal.

It's important to keep the tea-and-lye mixture as cold as possible, so you may need to change out the cold-water bath as things heat up. This process should take 5 to 7 minutes. Heating the tea slowly by adding the lye slowly is key to keeping the color as neutral as possible. If using sodium lactate, add it to the lye mixture and stir to combine. Set aside until clear.

2. Melt and measure the coconut oil into a bowl large enough to hold all the oils and the lye mixture. Add the shea butter to the hot coconut oil, and stir until it is melted. If needed, heat in 10-second bursts in the microwave, stirring between bursts until the butter melts. Add the olive oil pure and canola oil to the hot oils.

3. When the oils and the lye mixture are both below 110°F (43°C), add the lye mixture to the oils, pouring it over a spatula or the shaft of the stick blender to minimize air bubbles. Tap the stick blender a couple of times against the bottom of the bowl to release any air that may be trapped in the blades. *Do not turn on the stick blender until it is fully immersed.* Stick-blend for 30 seconds, or until very light trace is achieved. Add all of the eucalyptus essential oil, and stick-blend for another 5 seconds to combine.

4. Divide the batch into two containers:
  » Container A: 1 tablespoon titanium dioxide mixture
  » Container B: ¾ tablespoon green chrome mixture

Stick blend each container for 5 seconds. Pour into squirt bottles.

POUR THE SOAP

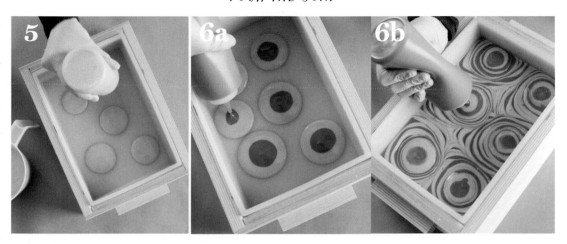

5. Squirt white circles into the mold in a random pattern. Count to 5 as you squeeze, to help keep the circles in similar sizes. We had 6 circles in our mold to start with.

6. Squirt green soap directly in the center of each white circle, again counting to 5 for each squirt. You want the soap to squirt into the previous circle, so don't be afraid to squirt firmly. Repeat the process, alternating with green and white soap. Tamp the mold down often to settle the soap. Do not use dividers in this soap, or it will disrupt the design.

FINAL STEPS

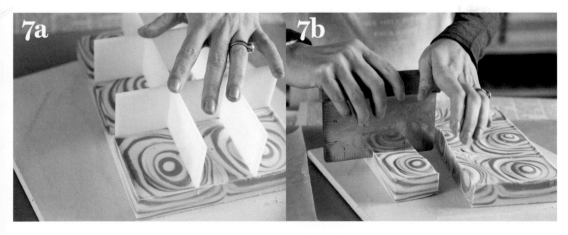

7. Allow the soap to set for at least 48 hours before unmolding, then cut into bars. You can use the divider set as a guide to cut even bars.

8. Allow the bars to cure in a well-ventilated area for 4 to 6 weeks before using, turning them every few days to ensure that they cure evenly.

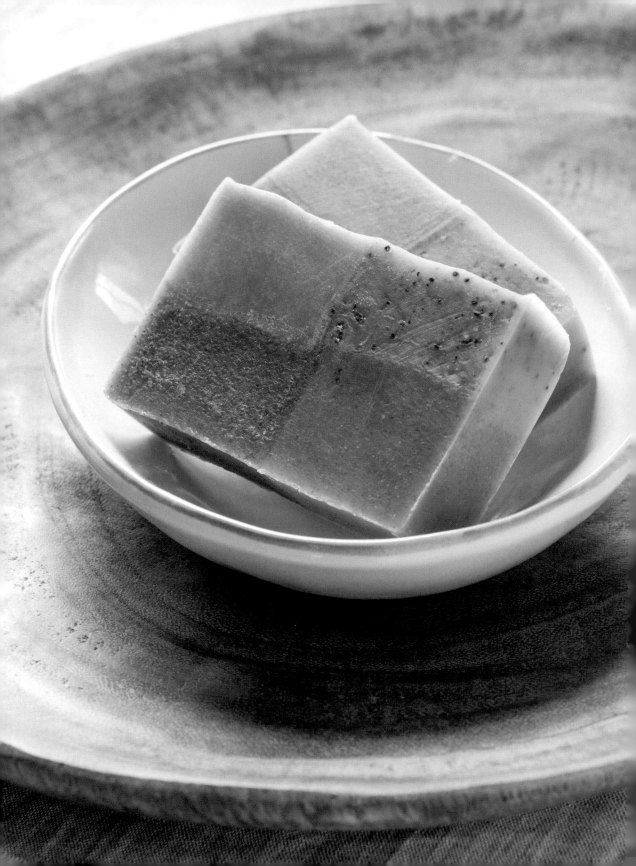

Gardener Scrub

with
COFFEE GROUNDS

Approximately 20 bars

The perfect soap for cleaning up after working outside, this super-scrubby bar gets the dirt off your fingers while leaving behind a fresh, herbaceous scent. For extra exfoliation, use large grounds; for gentler soap, use a finer grind.

Easy-pour containers with long spouts are highly recommended for this project; they allow you to get close to the soap while pouring layers in the small spaces between the dividers. Gel phase will help the colors in this recipe pop.

Mold and Special Tools

- » 5-pound wooden mold with sliding bottom with silicone liner
- » Multi-pour sectioning tool
- » Heating pad

Lye-Water Amounts

- 6.9 ounces lye (5% superfat)
- 16.5 ounces distilled water
- 1 1/2 tablespoons sodium lactate (optional)

Oil Amounts

- 10 ounces palm oil (20%)
- 12.5 ounces coconut oil (25%)
- 2.5 ounces avocado butter (5%)
- 17.5 ounces olive oil pure (35%)
- 7.5 ounces canola oil (15%)

Essential Oil Blend

- 1.5 ounces lemongrass essential oil
- 1 ounce rosemary essential oil
- 0.5 ounce basil essential oil

Colorant and Additive Amounts

- 5 teaspoons paprika dispersed into 1 tablespoon of canola oil
- 5 teaspoons ground orange peel dispersed into 1 tablespoon of canola oil
- 5 teaspoons brewed coffee grounds
- 10 teaspoons green zeolite clay dispersed into 2 tablespoons distilled water
- 2 teaspoons spirulina dispersed into 2 tablespoons canola oil

Safe Soaping!

Wear proper safety gear the whole time.

Work in a well-ventilated space.

No distractions (keep kids and pets away).

MAKE THE SOAP MIXTURE

1. Add the lye to the water (never the other way around) and stir gently until all of the lye is dissolved. If using sodium lactate, add it to the lye-water and stir to combine. Set the mixture aside to cool until it becomes clear.

2. Melt the palm oil in its original container, mix it thoroughly, and measure into a bowl large enough to hold all of the oils and the lye-water with room for mixing. Melt and measure the coconut oil and add it to the bowl. Add the avocado butter, and stir it in the hot oils until the butter is melted. Add the olive oil pure and the canola oil.

3. When both the oils and the lye-water are between 110° and 120°F (43–49°C), add the lye-water to the oils, pouring it over a spatula or the shaft of the stick blender to minimize air bubbles. Tap the stick blender a couple of times against the bottom of the bowl to release any air that may be trapped in the blades. *Do not turn on the stick blender until it is fully immersed.* Stick-blend for 30 seconds, or until very light trace is achieved.

4. Set up the mold with one long divider down the middle, pushed firmly to the bottom. Use a cross-section divider just across the top of the mold to hold the long one centered while you pour.

COLOR THE SOAP

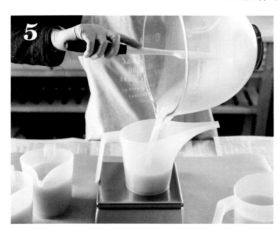

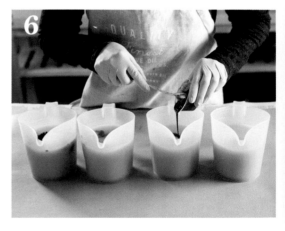

5. Divide the batter into four exactly equal sections. If you trust your visual skills, you can measure this way, or you can weigh the batter as you pour it into each container. Each container should have approximately 20 ounces by weight of soap batter.

6. Add the following amounts to the containers:
   » Container A: All of the paprika dispersion
   » Container B: All of the orange peel powder
   » Container C: All of the coffee grounds
   » Container D: All of the zeolite clay, 1 teaspoon of the spirulina powder dispersion

Stick-blend each container for 15 seconds, making sure to incorporate all of the colorants fully. Whisk about one-fourth of the essential oil into each container.

POUR THE SOAP

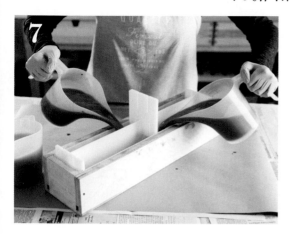

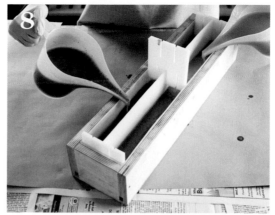

7. For the first layer, slowly pour the green zeolite and the paprika soap on opposite sides of the divider, at an even rate. Gently tap the mold on the table to settle once all of the soap is poured.

8. Next, pour the second layer. Move the spout of the containers as close to the first layer as possible to avoid breaking through. Pour the coffee soap over the paprika soap, and the orange peel soap over the spirulina soap.

FINAL STEPS

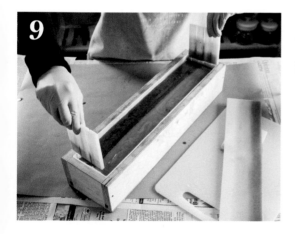

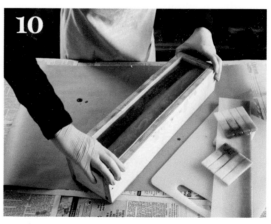

9. Pull the divider straight up out of the soap, and then gently remove the end pieces. Spritz with 99% rubbing alcohol to help prevent soda ash. Cover the mold with a towel and place it on a heating pad for 30 minutes to encourage gel phase.

10. Allow the soap to harden for 48 hours before attempting to unmold, then cut into bars. To remove the sliding bottom, turn the entire mold on its side and pull the bottom out. Allow the bars to cure in a well-ventilated area for 4 to 6 weeks before using, turning them every few days to ensure that they cure evenly.

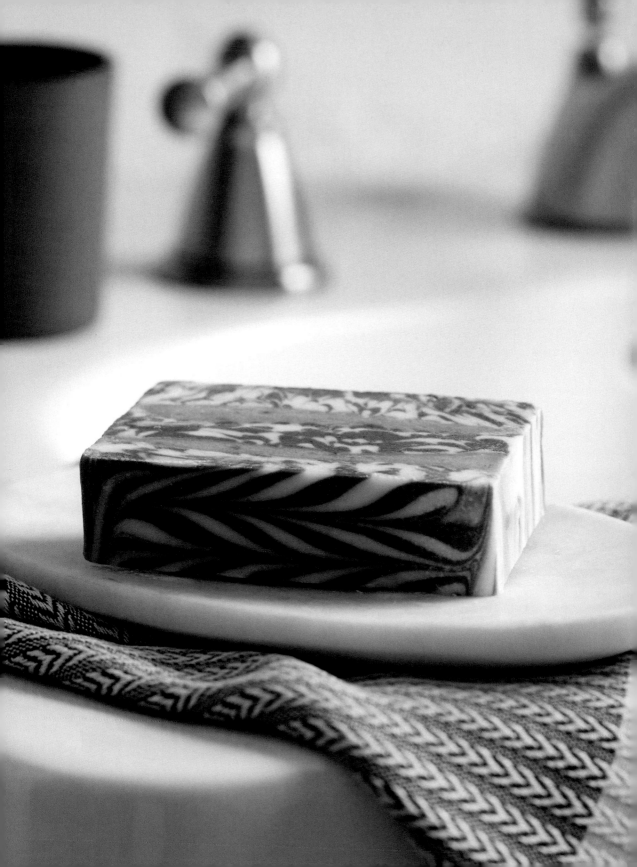

Layered Tomato
SWIRL BARS

Approximately 12 bars

Tomatoes may seem like a surprising ingredient in a soap, but their beautiful, rich color hints at skin-loving nutrients, such as lycopene, which is thought to help with the effects of aging. The tea tree and peppermint essential oils in this recipe leave a refreshing, cooling feeling on the skin. The contrasting colors and bold layers make an eye-catching design.

Mold and Special Tools

- » 10-inch silicone loaf mold
- » 2 squirt bottles
- » Chopstick or similar swirling tool

Lye-Water Amounts

- 4.6 ounces lye (5% superfat)
- 10.9 ounces distilled water
- 1 tablespoon sodium lactate (optional)

Oil Amounts

- 9.9 ounces coconut oil (30%)
- 3.3 ounces mango butter (10%)
- 8.2 ounces canola oil (25%)
- 9.9 ounces olive oil pomace (30%)
- 1.6 ounces hazelnut oil (5%)

Colorant and Additive Amounts

- 2 teaspoons activated charcoal dispersed into 2 tablespoons canola oil
- 1.5 ounces tomato paste

Essential Oil Blend

- 0.7 ounce peppermint 2nd distilled essential oil
- 0.7 ounce tea tree essential oil

Safe Soaping!

Wear proper safety gear the whole time.

Work in a well-ventilated space.

No distractions (keep kids and pets away).

MAKE THE SOAP MIXTURE

1. Slowly add the lye to the distilled water (never the other way around) and stir gently until all of the lye is dissolved. If using sodium lactate, add it to the lye-water and stir to combine. Set the mixture aside to cool until it becomes clear.

2. Melt the coconut oil in its original container, and measure into a bowl large enough to hold all of the oils and the lye-water with room for mixing. Add the mango butter to the hot oil, and stir until melted. If needed, heat the coconut/mango butter in 15-second bursts in the microwave to melt completely. Add the canola oil, olive oil pomace, and hazelnut oil to the hot oils.

3. When both the lye and the oils have cooled to between 110° and 120°F (43–49°C), slowly pour the lye-water into the oils, pouring it over a spatula or the shaft of the stick blender to minimize air bubbles. Tap the stick blender a couple of times against the bottom of the bowl to release any air that may be trapped in the blades. *Do not turn on the stick blender until it is fully immersed.* Stick-blend for 25 seconds, or until very light trace is achieved. Add all of the essential oil, and whisk to combine.

4. Separate the batter into three separate containers. Add the following colorants to the containers:

> » Container A: 1.5 tablespoons activated charcoal dispersion
> » Container B: 1.5 ounces tomato paste
> » Container C: Uncolored (white)

5. Stick-blend each container (moving from lightest to darkest) for 5 seconds to incorporate the color. Pour the black and the white batter (Containers A and C) into squirt bottles.

POUR AND SWIRL

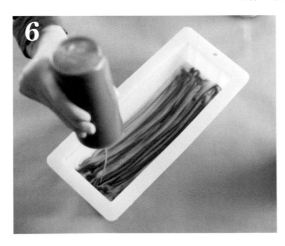

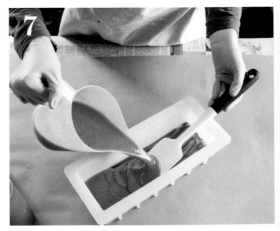

6. Begin the pattern by squirting stripes of black and white lengthwise across the bottom of the mold, alternating colors. Continue until you have approximately a ½-inch layer of soap. Tamp the mold to release any bubbles.

7. Pour the tomato paste soap over the back of a spatula over the striped soap. Pour low and slow to avoid breaking through the layers. Use half of the tomato paste soap for this layer.

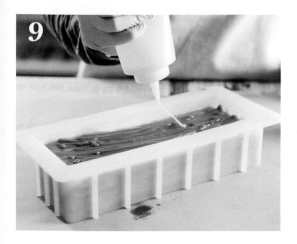

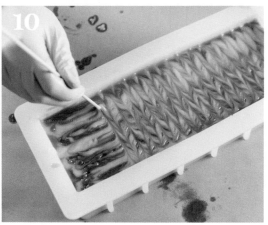

8. Repeat steps 6 and 7.

9. After the second layer of tomato soap has been poured, continue making straight lines of the black and white soap until all soap has been used.

10. Insert the swirling tool about ¼ inch into the soap in one corner. Working down the length of the mold, drag the tool from one side of the mold to the other to create narrow U shapes perpendicular to the lines of soap.

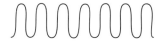

FINAL STEPS

11. Spray the surface of the soap with 99% rubbing alcohol to help prevent soda ash, and cover the soap while it rests. Allow it to sit undisturbed for 48 to 72 hours before attempting to unmold.

12. Once unmolded, cut the soap into bars and leave them in a well-ventilated area to cure for 4 to 6 weeks before using, turning them every few days to ensure that they cure evenly.

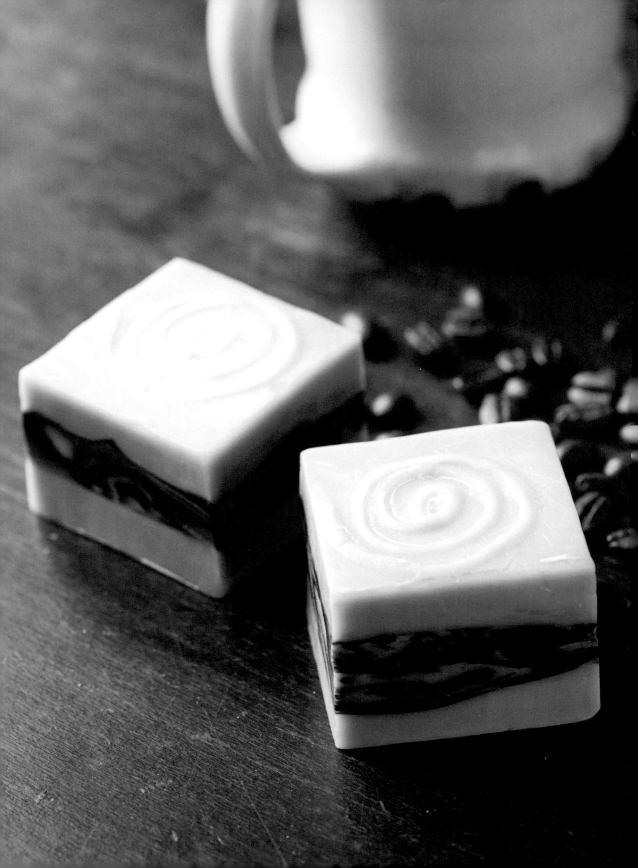

Coffee Swirl
LAYERED CUBES

Approximately 9 bars

A cup of coffee is usually known for waking you up in the morning, but caffeine also provides a jolt for your skin. It is a popular ingredient in some anti-cellulite creams. The rich, warm scent of the balsam Peru essential oil and the creamy tan color imparted from the brewed coffee make this soap smell and look almost good enough to eat. I fell in love with the beautiful "reverse stamp" technique on Auntie Clara's Handcrafted Cosmetics blog and have recreated it for you here. There are many options for creating your own stamp designs.

Mold and Special Tools

- » 6-inch silicone slab mold
- » 10-inch length of 19-gauge (or similar) stainless steel wire bent into a 1½-inch-diameter spiral

Lye-Water Amounts

- 3.0 ounces lye (5% superfat)
- 7.2 ounces cooled coffee
- 2 teaspoons sodium lactate (optional)

Oil Amounts

- 7.5 ounces olive oil pomace (34%)
- 5 ounces rice bran oil (23%)
- 0.6 ounce castor oil (3%)
- 1.1 ounces coffee butter (5%)
- 2.2 ounces cocoa butter (10%)
- 5.5 ounces coconut oil (25%)

Colorant

- 1 teaspoon activated charcoal mixed in 1 tablespoon rice bran oil

Essential Oil

- 1 ounce balsam Peru essential oil

Safe Soaping!

Wear proper safety gear the whole time.

Work in a well-ventilated space.

No distractions (keep kids and pets away).

MAKE THE SOAP MIXTURE

1. Slowly add the lye to the cooled coffee, stirring constantly until the lye is dissolved. As the lye reacts with the coffee, it will turn a green hue and produce a distinctive smell. This smell is normal, and will dissipate in the finished soap. Once all of the lye flakes are dissolved, stir in the sodium lactate (if using) and set aside to cool.

2. In a bowl large enough to hold all the oils and the lye-coffee solution, measure out the olive oil pomace, rice bran oil, and castor oil. In a separate container, measure out and melt the coffee butter, cocoa butter, and coconut oil in 20-second bursts to avoid overheating. Once the butters are completely melted, combine with the liquid oils in the large container.

3. When both the oils and the lye-mixture are between 110° and 120°F (43–49°C), add the coffee-lye solution to the oils, pouring it over a spatula or the shaft of the stick blender to minimize air bubbles. Tap the stick blender a couple of times against the bottom of the bowl to release any air that may be trapped in the blades. *Do not turn on the stick blender until it is fully immersed.* Stick-blend for 50 seconds, or until thin trace is achieved.

4. Add all of the essential oil, and stick-blend again for 15 seconds.

ADD COLORANTS

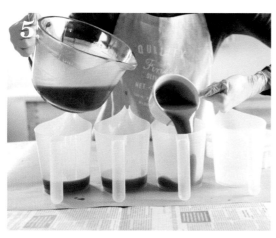 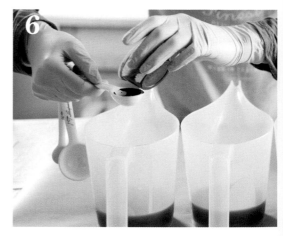

5. Split the batch into four easy-pour containers with the following amounts:
> » Container A: 1 ¼ cups (300ml)
> » Container B: 1 ¼ cups (300ml)
> » Container C: ⅔ cup (150ml)
> » Container D: ⅔ cup (150ml)

6. To Container C, add 2 teaspoons of the activated charcoal dispersion.

POUR, SWIRL, AND STAMP

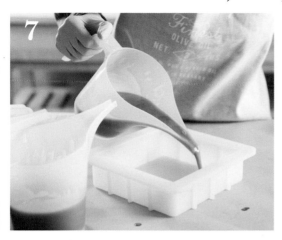

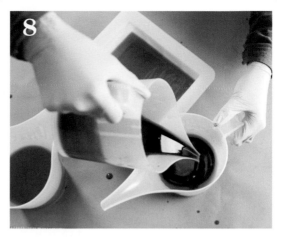

7. Blend Container A (uncolored batter) with the stick blender for 5 seconds. Pour all of this batter into the mold, and tap the mold on the table until smooth.

8. Pour the black batter (Container C) in a spiral pattern into the small uncolored batch of soap (Container D). Pour from at least 6 inches above the container so the black penetrates all the way through the uncolored soap.

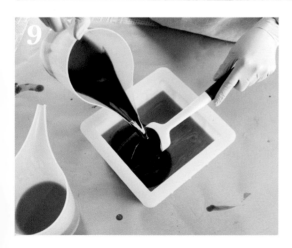

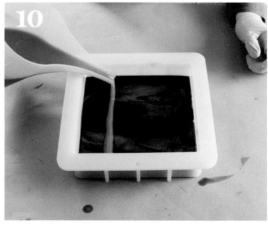

9. Slowly pour the black and tan swirl from Container D over the first layer of soap. Pour over the back of a spatula, and as low to the first layer as possible to avoid breaking the first layer. Pour the entire swirled mixture.

10. Whisk the soap in container B to loosen the batter. Again pouring low and slow, or over the back of a spatula, pour about half of the batter carefully over the swirled layer.

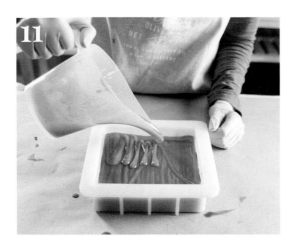

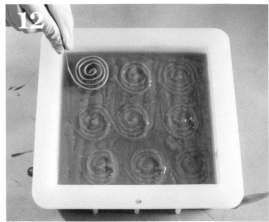

11. Stick blend the remaining batter in container B for about 10 seconds. Carefully pour the thickened soap into the mold, and gently tamp the mold to settle the batter.

12. Insert the wire tool just under the surface of the soap, in one corner. When you pull it up, it should draw the soap into a spiral design with it. If the soap is too thin to hold the pattern, let it sit for 5 more minutes and try again. Repeat the pattern across the surface of the soap in three rows of three.

FINAL STEPS

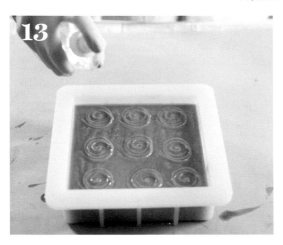

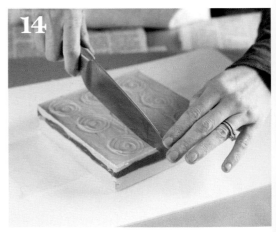

13. Spritz the soap with 99% rubbing alcohol, and allow the soap to set for 48 hours before attempting to unmold. If it is not releasing from the mold, let it set another 24 hours, or place it in the freezer for 3 hours and try again.

14. Cut the slab into bars. Allow the bars to cure in a well-ventilated area for 4 to 6 weeks before using, turning them every few days to ensure that they cure evenly.

Alkanet Layers
WITH PENCIL LINES

Approximately 12 bars

Alkanet root produces a beautiful array of colors from light gray to deep lavender. It is amazing to watch the color change as the brilliant magenta infusion hits the alkaline soap and transforms into purple before your eyes! The multiple pencil lines and angled pours add to the visual interest of the final bars. The color of alkanet root is enhanced by heat, so don't skip the gel phase on this soap (see What Is Gel Phase?, page 32).

Mold and Special Tools

- » 10-inch silicone loaf mold
- » 1-inch-thick notebook or similar item to tip the mold
- » Powder duster

Lye-water Amounts

4.6 ounces lye (5% superfat)

10.8 ounces distilled water

1 tablespoon sodium lactate (optional)

Oil Amounts

9.9 ounces palm oil (30%)

8.3 ounces coconut oil (25%)

11.6 ounces olive oil pomace (35%)

3.3 ounces refined hempseed oil (10%)

Essential Oil Blend

1.1 ounces lavender 40/42 essential oil*

0.4 ounce fennel essential oil

Colorant and Additive Amounts

- 2 teaspoons titanium dioxide dispersed into 2 tablespoons hemp oil
- 2 tablespoons alkanet root powder infused in 2 ounces olive oil pomace**
- 1 tablespoon alkanet root powder, dry

Regular lavender essential oil will work, but this variety has been specifically blended to last in cold-process soap.

**See pages 48–49 for instructions on infusing herbs.*

> *Note:* Each layer in this soap is thickened individually to avoid having the entire batch get too thick. While there are only two colors, you will need four containers to achieve this technique.

Safe Soaping!

Wear proper safety gear the whole time.

Work in a well-ventilated space.

No distractions (keep kids and pets away).

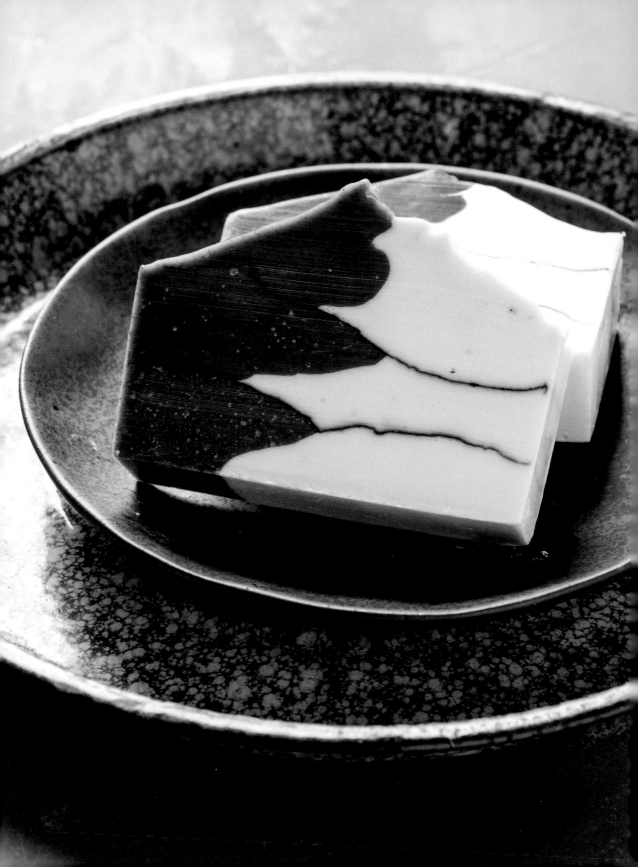

MAKE THE SOAP MIXTURE

1. Add the lye to the water (never the other way around) and stir gently until all of the lye is dissolved. If using sodium lactate, add it to the lye-water and stir to combine. Set the mixture aside to cool until it becomes clear.

2. Melt the palm oil in its original container, mix it thoroughly, and measure into a bowl large enough to hold all of the oils and the lye-water with room for mixing. Melt and measure the coconut oil and add it to the bowl. Add the olive oil pomace and refined hempseed oil.

3. When both the oils and lye-water are between 120° and 130°F (49–54°C), add the lye-water to the oils, pouring it over a spatula or the shaft of the stick blender to minimize air bubbles. Tap the stick blender a couple of times against the bottom of the bowl to release any air that may be trapped in the blades. *Do not turn on the stick blender until it is fully immersed.* Stick-blend for 20 seconds, or until trace is just reached. Add the essential oil blend, and whisk to combine.

4. Divide the batter equally between two containers. Add the following and whisk to combine.

» Container A: 2 tablespoons titanium dioxide mixture

» Container B: 2 ounces alkanet root infusion

5. Pour off just over 1 cup of batter from each color into two more easy-pour containers: white soap in Container C and purple soap in Container D.

POUR THE SOAP

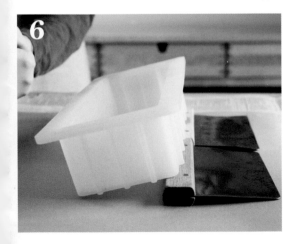

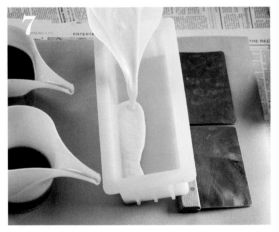

6. Set the mold up with one long side resting on the notebook or other wedge.

7. Stick-blend the white batter in Container C for 5 seconds, or until medium trace is reached. Pour this batter into the lower side of the tipped mold.

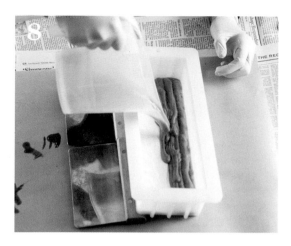

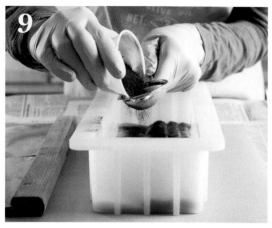

8. Stick-blend the purple batter in Container D for 5 seconds, or until medium trace is reached. Gently switch the wedge to the other side of the mold, so it is resting under the first layer of soap.

Pour the purple soap (Container D) into the lower side of the mold, beside the white layer.

9. Place a teaspoon of alkanet powder into the powder duster, and gently tap the duster over top of the soap until there is a light dusting of powder across the entire surface.

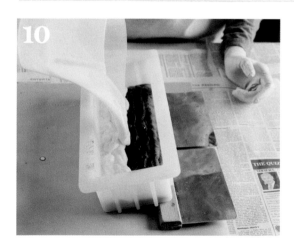

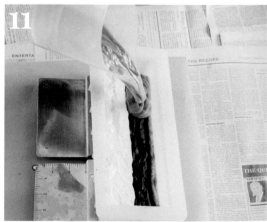

10. Pour another cup of batter into containers C and D from containers A and B with their respective colors. Stick-blend containers C and D for 5 seconds or until medium trace is reached.

Switch the wedge under the mold again, and gently pour a layer of thickened white soap into the lower edge, over the first white layer.

11. Allow the white layer to set for 10 seconds, and switch the wedge again. Pour 1 cup of thickened purple over the first purple layer.

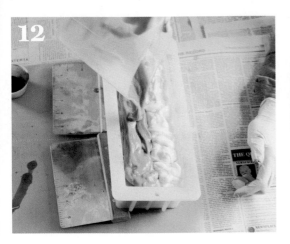

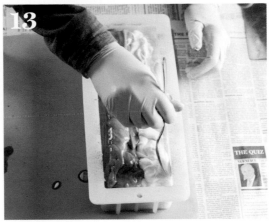

12. Repeat steps 9 through 11 with the remaining two containers, thickening the batter as needed, until all of the soap is gone.

13. Using the back of a spoon, gently pull the sides of the soap batter from the outer edge, to the center, building it into a peak. Clean off the spoon between the purple and the white sides so you do not blend colors.

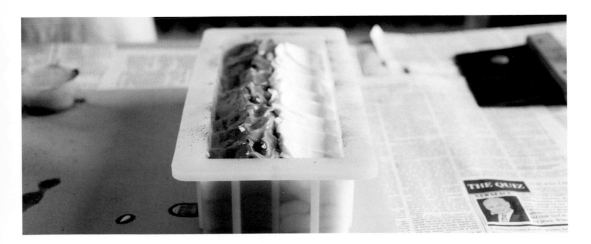

FINAL STEPS

14. Cover and insulate the mold. Place it on a heating pad on medium for 1 hour. Turn off the heating pad, leaving the covered mold on it. Allow it to set for 72 hours.

15. Once out of the mold, cut the soap on its side to help avoid drag marks from the pencil lines. Allow the bars to cure in a well-ventilated area for 4 to 6 weeks before using, turning them every few days to ensure that they cure evenly.

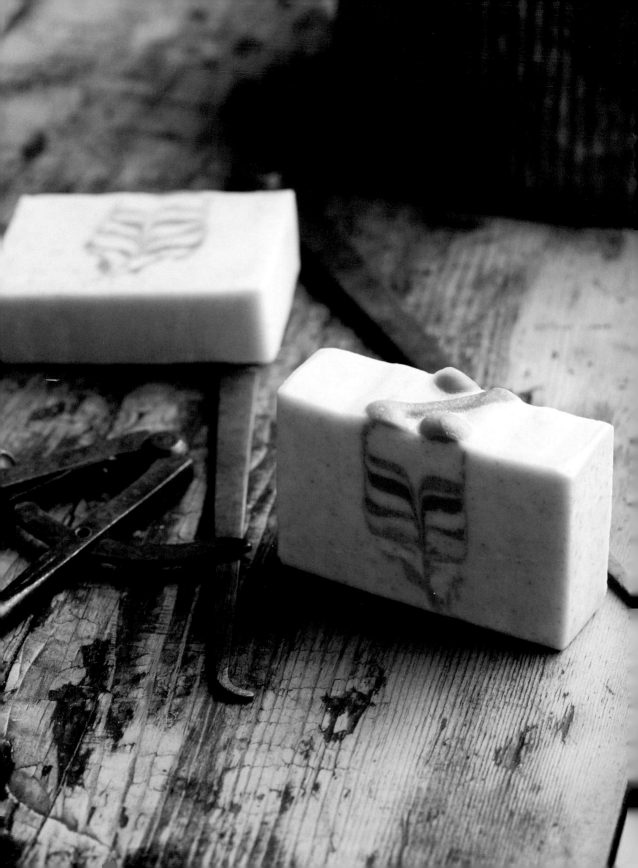

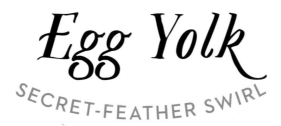

Egg Yolk
SECRET-FEATHER SWIRL

Approximately 20 bars

Everyone knows eggs are a beneficial food, but it's less commonly known that they can be used in skincare. This recipe uses just the nutrient-packed yolk, which contains vitamins A and B_3. The design of this soap may look simple, but it is not for the faint of heart! To get the best effect, keep the trace nice and thin to give yourself time to create all the layers.

Mold and Special Tools

- » 5-pound sliding bottom log mold with silicone liner
- » Multi-pour sectioning tool
- » Powder duster (or similar thin mesh strainer)
- » 4 (8-ounce) squirt bottles
- » Wire hanger and plastic drinking straws to make swirling tool

Lye-Water Amounts

8.4 ounces lye (5% superfat)

19.8 ounces distilled water

1¼ tablespoons sodium lactate (optional)

Oil Amounts

14.4 ounces palm oil (24%)

14.4 ounces coconut oil (24%)

1.8 ounces avocado butter (3%)

1.2 ounces palm kernel flakes (2%)

1.8 ounces castor oil (3%)

3 ounces sweet almond oil (5%)

10.2 ounces canola oil (17%)

9.2 ounces olive oil pure* (22%)

Essential Oil Blend

2 ounces lavender 40/42 essential oil**

0.5 ounces litsea cubeba essential oil

Colorant and Additive Amounts

- 1 teaspoon ultramarine pink oxide dispersed into 1 tablespoon sweet almond oil
- 2 teaspoons titanium dioxide dispersed into 2 tablespoons sweet almond oil
- 1 teaspoon black oxide dispersed into 1 tablespoon sweet almond oil
- 1 teaspoon chrome green oxide dispersed into 1 tablespoon sweet almond oil
- 4 egg yolks, room temperature
- 4 ounces olive oil pure

*Plus 4 ounces mixed with the egg yolks and added at trace, for a total of 13.2 ounces

**Regular lavender essential oil will work, but this variety has been specifically blended to last in cold-process soap.

Safe Soaping!

Wear proper safety gear the whole time.

Work in a well-ventilated space.

No distractions (keep kids and pets away).

MAKE THE SWIRLING TOOL

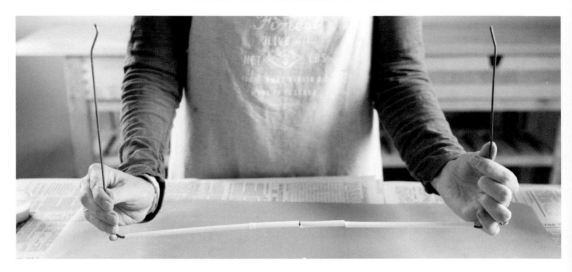

Untwist the hooked end of a wire hanger. Pull the two ends apart to form an angled U shape with the long straight end as the base of the U. Measure the straight end of the hanger alongside the long end of the mold. Use a pair of needle-nose pliers to bend the hanger to fit inside the mold. Thread plastic drinking straws onto the straight bottom of the hanger, cutting them to fit across the entire length. This makes a thicker line that creates a more dramatic feather effect.

MAKE THE SOAP MIXTURE

1. Add the lye to the water (never the other way around) and stir gently until all of the lye is dissolved. If using sodium lactate, add it to the lye-water and stir to combine. Set the mixture aside to cool until it becomes clear.

2. Melt the palm oil in its original container, mix it thoroughly, and measure into a bowl large enough to hold all of the oils and the lye-water with room for mixing. Melt the coconut oil, and add the avocado butter and palm kernel flakes to the hot oils, and stir until melted. If needed, microwave in 10-second bursts. Add the castor oil, sweet almond oil, canola oil, and 9.2 ounces of the olive oil pure to the rest of the oils.

3. In a small cup, combine the remaining 4 ounces of olive oil pure with the egg yolks.

4. Temperatures are important in this recipe; you don't want to "cook" the egg in the oil. When the oils and lye-water are between 85° and 95°F (29–35°C), add the lye-water to the oils, pouring it over a spatula or the shaft of the stick blender to minimize air bubbles. Tap the stick blender a couple of times against the bottom of the bowl to release any air that may be trapped in the blades. *Do not turn on the stick blender until it is fully immersed.* Stick-blend for 20 seconds, or until very thin trace is achieved.

5. Pour the egg yolk and oil mixture into the bowl through a strainer. Combine with a whisk.

6. Pour slightly less than ½ cup (115ml) of batter into three easy-pour containers, leaving the bulk of the batter in the bowl.

7. Add the following colors to the containers:
- » Main batter: 1½ tablespoons titanium dioxide dispersion
- » Container A: 1 teaspoon ultramarine pink dispersion
- » Container B: ½ teaspoon titanium dioxide dispersion, 1 teaspoon ultramarine pink dispersion, ¹/₁₆ teaspoon black dispersion
- » Container C: ¼ teaspoon green chrome dispersion

8. Add all of the essential oil to the main batch of soap, and stick-blend for 5 seconds. Split off 2 cups of this white batter, and set aside.

POUR INTO DIVIDERS

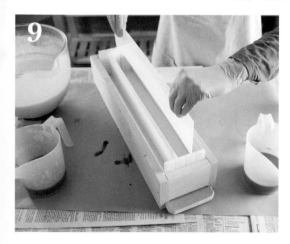

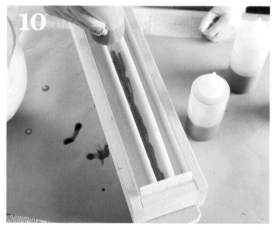

9. Pour a ½-inch layer of the main soap into the mold. Insert the multi-pour sectioning tool with the three-section option (two dividers) directly into the soap.

10. Fill the squirt bottles, one with pink batter, one with green batter, one with purple batter, and one with white batter (from the main batch, not the 2-cup batch).

Squirt a layer of green batter in the center section of the divider set. The green will not completely cover the white layer; it is okay to have gaps showing through.

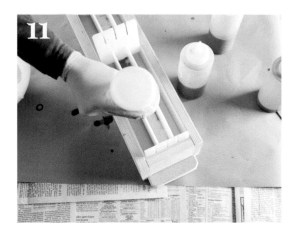

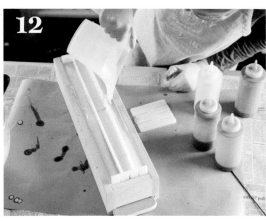

11. Squirt a layer of white batter over the green layer. Again, full coverage is not required.

Squirt more layers in the center section in the following pattern:

- » Green
- » White
- » Purple
- » White

- » Pink
- » White
- » Purple
- » White

Refill the white squirt bottle as needed from the large batch of soap. Reserve about ⅛ cup of the green, pink, and purple soap batters.

12. Fill the outer dividers with the 2-cup batch white soap until each side reaches the depth of the soap in the center divider.

SWIRL THE SOAP

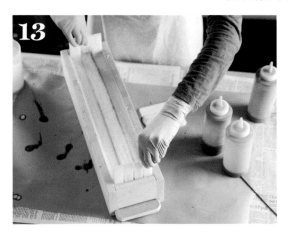

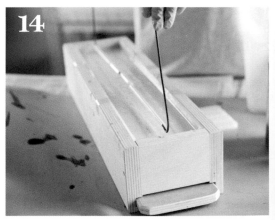

13. Carefully remove the two center dividers and then the pieces at each end, pulling straight up and out of the soap.

14. Insert the hanger tool straight down the middle of the colored soap to the bottom, through all the colored layers. Slide the tool along the bottom, up one side, and out of the soap.

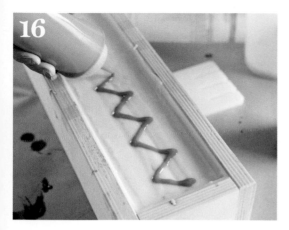

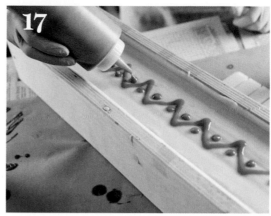

15. Whisk the white batter that was set aside in step 8. Gently pour it across the surface of the soap using a back-and-forth pattern. Pour all of the white batter for this step.

16. Using the leftover green batter, squirt a squiggle across the surface of the soap.

17. In each curve of the green squiggle, squirt a pink dot of soap. Squirt a smaller dot of purple on top of each pink dot.

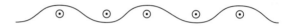

FINAL STEPS

18. Spritz the top of the soap with 99% rubbing alcohol, and allow it to set uncovered for 24 to 48 hours before attempting to unmold. To remove the sliding bottom, turn the entire mold on its side and pull the bottom out.

19. Cut into bars and allow them to cure in a well-ventilated area for 4 to 6 weeks before using, turning them every few days to ensure that they cure evenly.

CHAPTER 10

Colorful & Creative

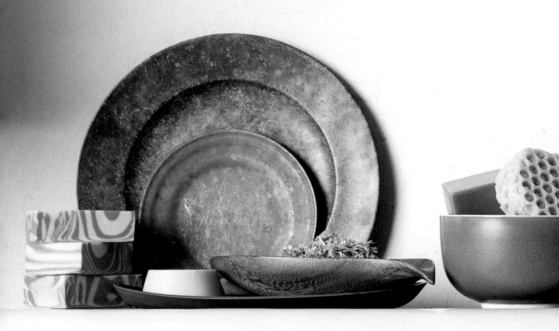

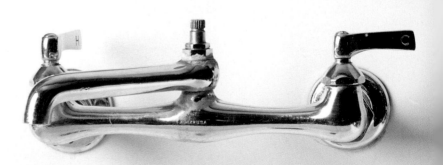

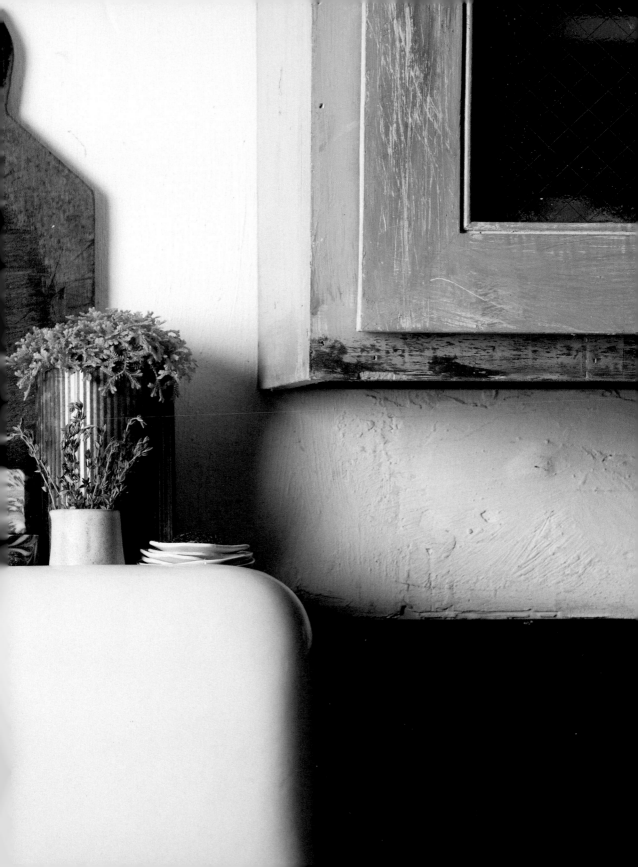

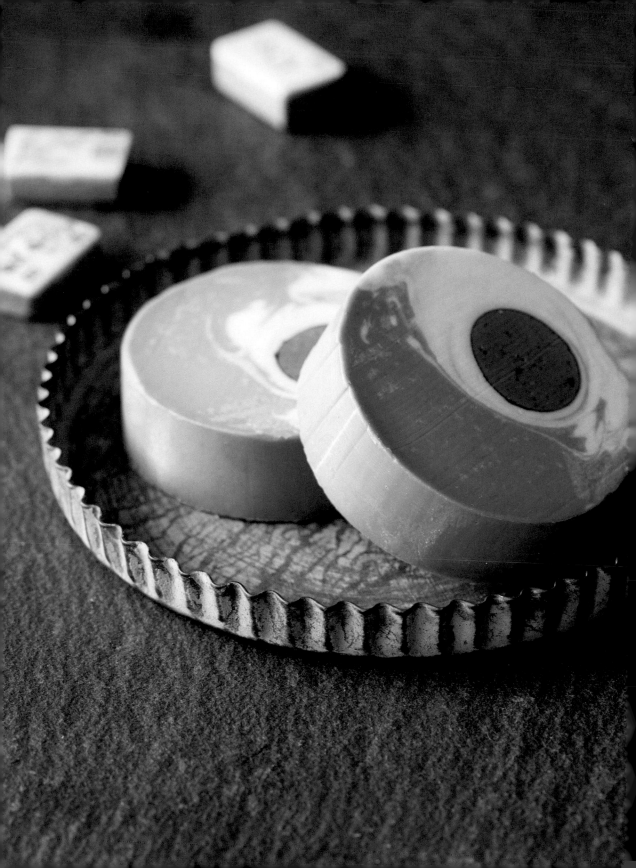

Blueberry Embed

ROUND BARS

Approximately 8 bars

This soap utilizes fresh blueberries and a high percentage of mango butter. Blueberries, a well-known superfood, are brimming with antioxidants that aid in fighting free radicals. Mango butter is rich in unsaponifiables, which means that many parts of this butter remain to moisturize the skin, and the high percentage of oleic acids make it a great humectant. The thin ring of activated charcoal really makes the blueberry embed pop!

STAGE 1
MAKE THE BLUEBERRY EMBED

Mold and Special Tools

» Mini round silicone column mold
» Powder duster

Lye-Water Amounts

0.7 ounce lye (5% superfat)
1.1 ounces distilled water
½ teaspoon sodium lactate (optional)

*Thaw first if using frozen.

Oil Amounts

1.5 ounces palm oil (30%)
1.5 ounces coconut oil (30%)
1.5 ounces olive oil pomace (30%)
0.5 ounce sweet almond oil (10%)

Essential Oil

0.1 ounce juniper berry essential oil

Colorant and Additive Amounts

10 whole blueberries*
1 teaspoon ultramarine blue dispersed into 1 tablespoon sweet almond oil
1 teaspoon titanium dioxide dispersed into 1 tablespoon sweet almond oil
1 teaspoon activated charcoal

Note: This beautiful design requires that the embeds cure for 48 hours before using them in the base soap, so plan ahead.

Safe Soaping!

Wear proper safety gear the whole time.

Work in a well-ventilated space.

No distractions (keep kids and pets away).

MAKE THE SOAP MIXTURE

1. Add the lye to the water (never the other way around) and stir gently until all of the lye is dissolved. If using sodium lactate, add it to the lye-water and stir to combine. Set the mixture aside to cool until it becomes clear.

2. Melt the palm oil in its original container, mix it thoroughly, and measure into a bowl large enough to hold all of the oils and the lye-water with room for mixing. Melt and measure the coconut oil and add it to the bowl. Add the olive oil pomace and sweet almond oil.

3. Add the blueberries to the oils, and stick-blend for 30 seconds on high. Try to get the blueberry skins as pureed as possible, with no chunks left.

4. When the oils and the lye-water are between 110° and 120°F (43–49°C), add the lye-water to the oils, pouring it over a spatula or the shaft of the stick blender to minimize air bubbles. Tap the stick blender a couple of times against the bottom of the bowl to release any air that may be trapped in the blades. *Do not turn on the stick blender until it is fully immersed.* Stick-blend for 10 seconds, or until thin trace is achieved.

MIX AND POUR

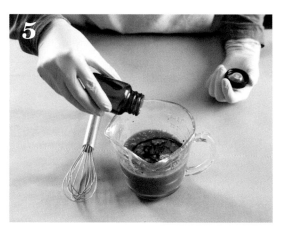

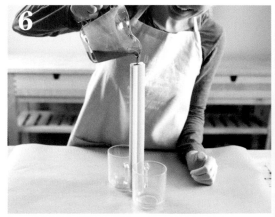

5. Add to the batter: 2 teaspoons ultramarine blue dispersion, ½ teaspoon titanium dioxide dispersion and all of the juniper essential oil.

6. Use a whisk to combine the colors and essential oil, and pour the batter into the silicone round mold. Prop the mold up with mugs or something similar to keep it stable. Let the soap sit for 24 to 48 hours before attempting to unmold. If sodium lactate was not used, allow the soap to cure for up to a week before unmolding.

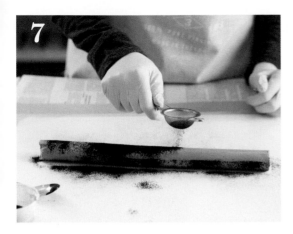

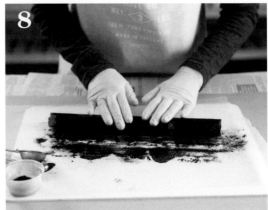

7. Place the unmolded soap on a newspaper or paper towel. Use the powder duster to sprinkle activated charcoal over the soap log.

8. Rub the powder along the log to spread the color evenly. Cover the entire outside of the embed, and gently tap it on its end to remove any loose powder.

STAGE 2
MAKE THE BACKGROUND SOAP

Mold and Special Tools
- » Silicone column mold
- » Two easy-pour containers

Lye-Water Amounts
- 2.6 ounces lye (5% superfat)
- 6.2 ounces distilled water
- 2 teaspoons sodium lactate (optional)

Oil Amounts
- 4.8 ounces palm oil (25%)
- 4.8 ounces coconut oil (25%)
- 1.9 ounces mango butter (10%)
- 2.9 ounces olive oil pure (15%)
- 4.8 ounces canola oil (25%)

Essential Oil Blend
- 0.5 ounce anise essential oil
- 0.5 ounce litsea essential oil

Colorant and Additive Amounts
- 1 teaspoon titanium dioxide dispersed into 1 tablespoon olive oil pure
- 1 teaspoon ultramarine blue dispersed into 1 tablespoon olive oil pure
- 1 blueberry embed soap (made 24–48 hours ahead of time)

MAKE THE SOAP MIXTURE

1. Add the lye to the water (never the other way around) and stir gently until all of the lye is dissolved. Add the sodium lactate to the lye-water and stir to combine. Set the mixture aside to cool until it becomes clear.

2. Melt the palm oil in its original container, mix it thoroughly, and measure into a bowl large enough to hold all of the oils and the lye-water with room for mixing. Melt and measure the coconut oil and add it to the bowl. Add the mango butter to the hot oils and stir until melted. If needed, place the oils and butter in the microwave in 10-second bursts until melted. Add the olive oil pure and canola oil.

3. When the oils and the lye-water are between 110° and 120°F (43–49°C), add the lye-water to the oils, pouring it over a spatula or the shaft of the stick blender to minimize air bubbles. Tap the stick blender a couple of times against the bottom of the bowl to release any air that may be trapped in the blades. *Do not turn on the stick blender until it is fully immersed.* Stick-blend for 20 seconds, or until thin trace is achieved.

4. Split the batter in half. Add the following colorants to each container:
  » Container A: 1 teaspoon titanium dioxide dispersion, half of the essential oil blend
  » Container B: 1 teaspoon ultramarine blue dispersion, ½ teaspoon titanium dioxide dispersion, half of the essential oil blend

POUR SOAP AND ADD EMBED

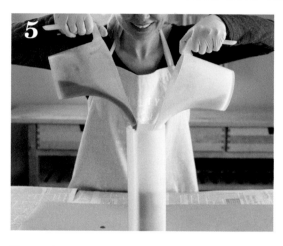

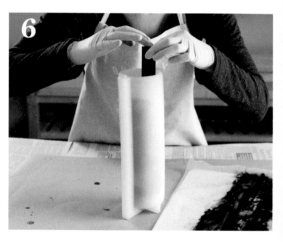

5. Simultaneously pour the blue and white batter into the mold until all of the batter is used.

6. Insert the blue soap embed straight into the soap batter, off-centered. Make sure it is not touching the sides of the mold.

FINISHING STEPS

7. Spritz the top of the mold with 99% rubbing alcohol to help avoid soda ash. Because this soap doesn't have very much surface area to "breathe," it needs to remain in the mold for at least 72 hours before you attempt to unmold it.

8. Once the soap is unmolded, cut it into bars. The activated charcoal tends to smear when first cut. To clean the bars up, let them dry out for about 2 days, then use the back of a knife to gently scrape off a very thin layer of soap. This should leave the lines looking clean and crisp.

Allow the bars to cure in a well-ventilated area for 4 to 6 weeks before using, turning them every few days to ensure that they cure evenly.

Charcoal Hearts

ROUND BARS

Approximately 8 bars

A ring of activated charcoal and a pattern of fun, colored embeds provide a striking contrast in this soap. The two-step process of creating embeds and a separate base soap is worth it for the stunning effect of the hearts against the swirled background.

STAGE 1
MAKE SOAP EMBEDS

Mold and Special Tools
- » 4 silicone heart embed molds
- » Cup or mug large enough to hold 4 molds upright

Lye-Water Amounts
- 2.1 ounces lye (5% superfat)
- 5.3 ounces distilled water
- 2 teaspoons sodium lactate (optional)

Oil Amounts
- 8.8 ounces lard (55%)
- 2.4 ounces coconut oil (15%)
- 4.8 ounces olive oil pomace (30%)

Essential Oil Blend
- 0.8 ounce juniper berry essential oil
- 0.2 ounce clary sage essential oil

Colorants
- 2 teaspoons titanium dioxide dispersed into 2 tablespoons olive oil pomace
- 1 teaspoon ultramarine violet dispersed into 1 tablespoon olive oil pomace
- 1 teaspoon ultramarine pink oxide dispersed into 1 tablespoon olive oil pomace

Note: This beautiful design requires that the embeds cure for 48 hours before using them in the base soap, so plan ahead.

Safe Soaping!

Wear proper safety gear the whole time.

Work in a well-ventilated space.

No distractions (keep kids and pets away).

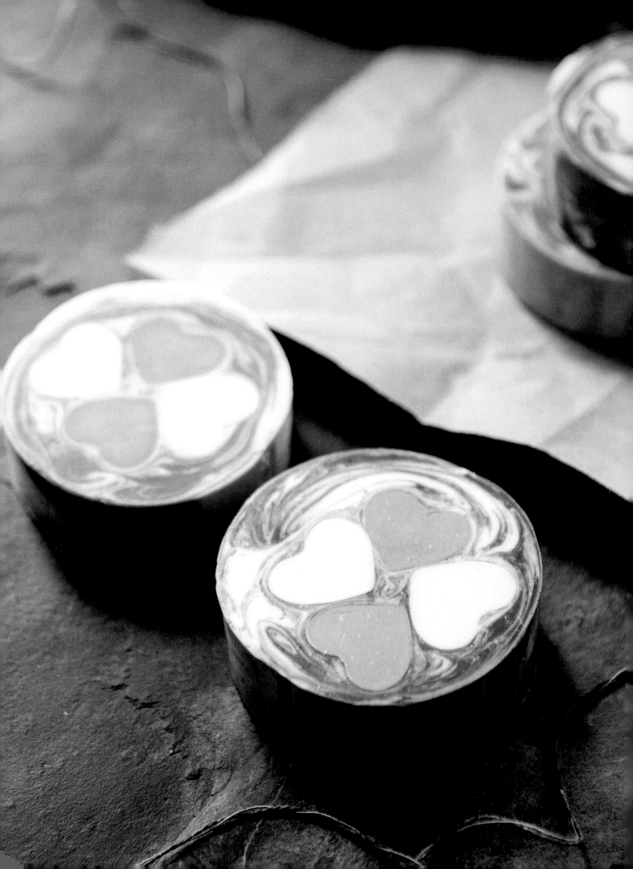

MAKE THE SOAP MIXTURE

1. Add the lye to the water (never the other way around) and stir gently until all of the lye is dissolved. If using sodium lactate, add it to the lye-water and stir to combine. Set the mixture aside to cool until it becomes clear.

2. In a bowl large enough to hold all the oils and the lye-water solution with room for mixing, measure out the lard and coconut oil. Microwave until both oils are liquid and clear. Measure out olive oil pomace, and combine with the melted oils.

3. When the oils and the lye-water are between 110° and 120°F (43–49°C), add the lye-water to the oils, pouring it over a spatula or the shaft of the stick blender to minimize air bubbles. Tap the stick blender a couple of times against the bottom of the bowl to release any air that may be trapped in the blades. *Do not turn on the stick blender until it is fully immersed.* Stick-blend for 10 seconds. Add all of the essential oil blend, and whisk to combine.

COLOR AND POUR

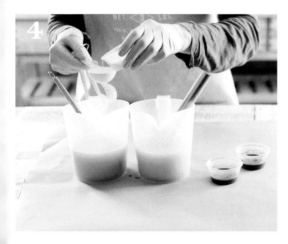 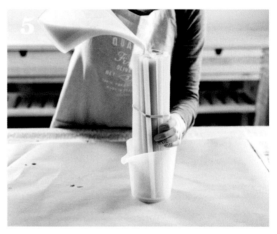

4. Divide the batter equally between two containers. Add the colorants as follows:
  » Container A: 1 tablespoon titanium dioxide dispersion
  » Container B: 2 teaspoons titanium dioxide dispersion, 2 teaspoons ultramarine violet dispersion, 2 teaspoons ultramarine pink dispersion

5. Balance the embed molds and make sure they are well supported (putting them in a container works well). Carefully pour the white batter into two of the molds (not next to each other) and the purple batter into the remaining ones.

6. Allow the soaps to harden for at least 48 hours before attempting to unmold. If needed, you can also put the hardened soaps in the freezer for 30 minutes to help ease the unmolding process.

STAGE 2

MAKE THE BASE SOAP

Mold

» Silicone column mold

Lye-water Amounts

2 ounces lye (5% superfat)

4.9 ounces distilled water

1 teaspoon sodium lactate (optional)

Oil Amounts

3.6 ounces olive oil pomace (24%)

3.8 ounces coconut oil (25%)

0.9 ounce cocoa butter (6%)

6.8 ounces lard (45%)

Essential Oil Blend

0.2 ounce clary sage essential oil

0.5 ounce juniper berry essential oil

Colorant and Additive Amounts

1 teaspoon activated charcoal dispersed into 1 tablespoon olive oil

1 teaspoon titanium dioxide dispersed into 1 tablespoon olive oil pure

4 heart embeds (made 24–48 hours ahead)

MAKE THE SOAP MIXTURE

1. Add the lye to the water (never the other way around) and stir gently until all of the lye is dissolved. Add 1 teaspoon sodium lactate to the lye-water and stir to combine. Set the mixture aside to cool until it becomes clear.

2. In a bowl large enough to hold all the oils and the lye-water solution with room for mixing, measure out the olive oil pomace. In a separate container, measure out and melt the coconut oil, cocoa butter, and lard. Once they are completely melted, combine with the olive oil in the large bowl.

3. When the oils and the lye-water are between 110° and 120°F (43–49°C), add the lye-water to the oils, pouring it over a spatula or the shaft of the stick blender to minimize air bubbles. Tap the stick blender a couple of times against the bottom of the bowl to release any air that may be trapped in the blades. *Do not turn on the stick blender until it is fully immersed.* Stick-blend for 15 seconds, or until very thin trace is achieved.

COLOR AND POUR

4. Split the batter into two equal portions. Add the following to each container:
  » Container A: 1 tablespoon titanium dioxide dispersion, half of the essential oil blend
  » Container B: 1 tablespoon activated charcoal dispersion, half of the essential oil blend

5. Stick-blend each container for 5 seconds to incorporate the color and essential oils.

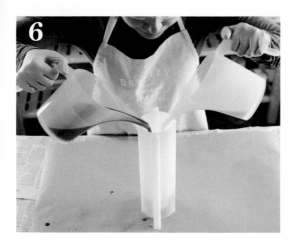

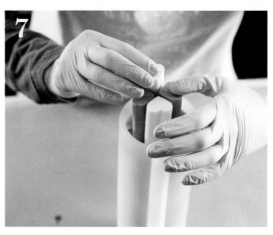

6. Simultaneously pour both soap batters into the silicone column mold, moving the containers around slightly to mix the colors (a horseshoe pattern works well). Use all of the batter for this step.

7. Insert the soap hearts one at a time into the soap batter, with the pointed end of each heart facing the center of the mold and touching to form a clover pattern.

FINAL STEPS

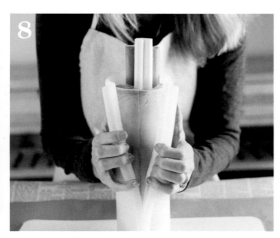

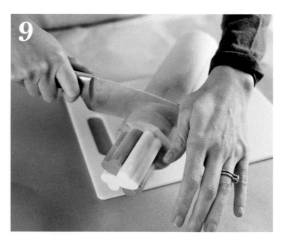

8. Spritz the top of the soap with 99% rubbing alcohol to help avoid soda ash. Let the soap set for 48 to 72 hours before attempting to unmold.

9. Once unmolded, cut into bars. Allow the bars to cure in a well-ventilated area for 4 to 6 weeks before using, turning them every few days to ensure that they cure evenly.

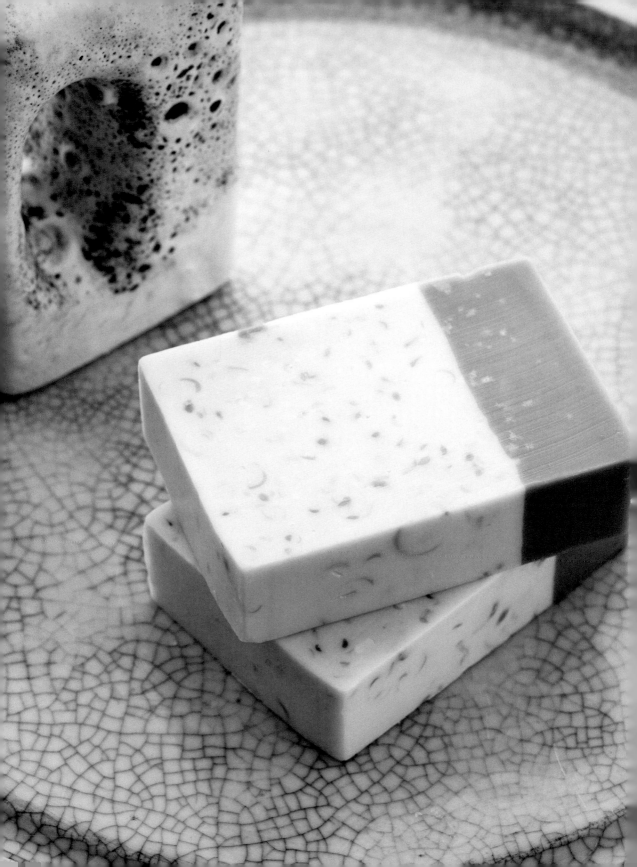

Almond Milk

CONFETTI BARS

Approximately 20 bars

Almond milk is full of nourishing vitamins E and B, which benefit dry skin. Elemi essential oil has been traditionally used to rejuvenate the skin, while rosemary is said to restore mental alertness. The delicate colors are visually enticing and the creamy lather of this soap in the shower is divine.

This recipe is soaped at cooler temperatures to prevent gel phase and keep the soap beautifully neutral (rather than brown) in color. Embedding soap shreds in this soap ensures that no soap goes to waste! You can use scraps or batches that didn't turn out how you planned, or create brightly colored soaps just for this recipe.

Mold and Special Tools

» 5-pound wooden mold with sliding bottom with silicone liner
» Multi-pour sectioning tool

Lye-Water Amounts

7.6 ounces lye (5% superfat)

18.1 ounces almond milk, frozen into cubes

5 teaspoons sodium lactate (optional)

Oil Amounts

11.6 ounces palm oil (21%)

13.8 ounces coconut oil (25%)

14.9 ounces olive oil pure (27%)

13.8 ounces rice bran oil (25%)

1.1 ounces castor oil (2%)

Essential Oil Blend

1.9 ounces elemi essential oil

0.6 ounce rosemary essential oil

Colorant and Additive Amounts

2 teaspoons ultramarine violet dispersed into 2 tablespoons rice bran oil

1 teaspoon titanium dioxide dispersed into 1 tablespoon rice bran oil

5 cups finely shredded leftover soaps in various colors

Safe Soaping!

Wear proper safety gear the whole time.

Work in a well-ventilated space.

No distractions (keep kids and pets away).

MAKE THE SOAP MIXTURE

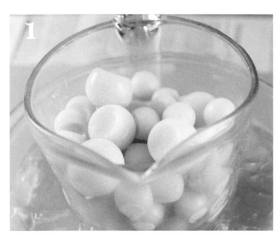

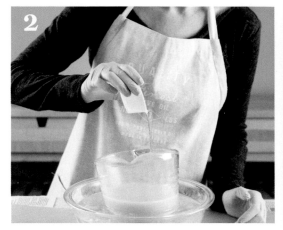

1. Measure the frozen almond milk into a heat-safe container. Place the container in a cold-water bath. Slowly and carefully pour about 1 tablespoon of the lye flakes over the almond milk. Stir for 2 minutes, then add another table-spoon. The more slowly the lye is added, the less the milk will discolor. Add 1 tablespoon at a time until all of the lye is dissolved and the cubes are melted. If using sodium lactate, add it to the lye-water and stir to combine. Set aside and allow the mixture to come to room temperature.

2. Melt the palm oil in its original container, mix thoroughly, and measure into a bowl large enough to hold all of the oils and the lye-water with room for mixing. Melt and measure the coconut oil and add it to the bowl. Add the olive oil pure, rice bran oil, and castor oil.

3. Once the oils are under 90°F (32°C), and the lye-milk mixture is between 60° and 70°F (15.5–21°C), slowly and carefully pour the lye into the oils. The natural fats in the almond milk may cause a few "floaties" in the lye-water. That is normal, and the chunks will be incorporated with the stick blender.

MIX AND POUR

4. Stick-blend the mixture for about 50 seconds, or until very thin trace is achieved. Portion out about 20 ounces of soap batter into a long-spouted, easy-pour container. Add all of the dispersed ultramarine violet to this container and stir with a whisk. To the large container of soap, add all of the dispersed titanium dioxide and stir it in with a whisk.

5. Stick-blend each container for 5 seconds to completely incorporate the colorants. Add two-thirds of the essential oil to the white batch of soap and the remaining one-third to the purple batch of soap and whisk to combine.

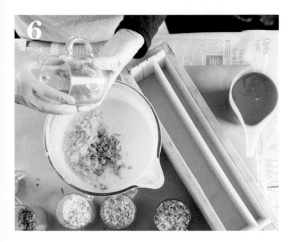

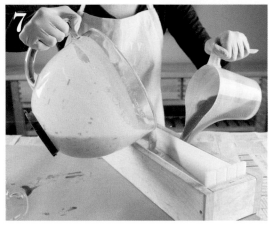

6. Using a single long divider, section the mold into two parts, about one third and two thirds of the total space. Add the shredded soap "confetti" to the white batch and stir it in with a spatula.

7. Simultaneously pour the purple soap into the small side of the mold and the white confetti soap into the larger side. Tap the mold firmly on the table to release any bubbles. Pull the center divider straight up and out of the soap.

FINAL STEPS

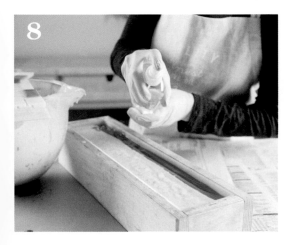

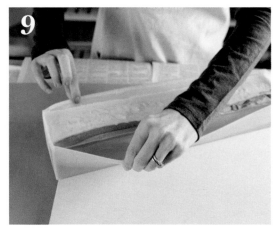

8. Spritz the soap with 99% rubbing alcohol, and place the entire mold in the freezer. Leave the soap in the freezer for about 8 to 12 hours, then allow it to thaw for another 24 hours before attempting to unmold.

9. Once unmolded, cut the soap into bars and allow them to cure in a well-ventilated area for 4 to 6 weeks before using, turning them every few days to ensure that they cure evenly.

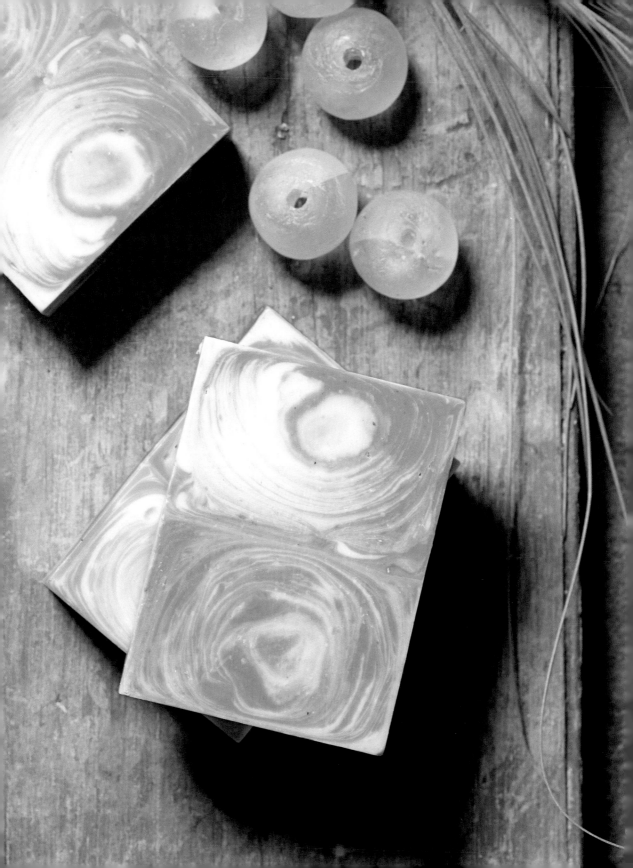

Tussah Silk

DOUBLE POUR

Approximately 16 bars

This luxurious bar incorporates real silk fibers, which create a rich lather and leave skin feeling smooth and soft. You may not want to make another batch of soap without silk after trying this one. The recipe also features green tea seed oil, a nourishing and exotic oil. A 20 percent water discount makes unmolding this soap from the dividers easier.

Mold

» Vertical wood mold with dividers

Lye-Water Amounts

6.1 ounces lye (5% superfat)

11.6 ounces distilled water (20% water discount)

4 teaspoons sodium lactate (optional)

Oil Amounts

11 ounces palm oil (25%)

11 ounces coconut oil (25%)

2.2 ounces avocado oil (5%)

8.8 ounces canola oil (20%)

2.2 ounces green tea seed oil (5%)

8.8 ounces olive oil pure (20%)

Essential Oil Blend

1.2 ounces lavender 40/42 essential oil*

0.8 ounce palmarosa essential oil

Additive Amounts

1 pinch tussah silk fibers

2 teaspoons titanium dioxide dispersed into 2 tablespoons avocado oil

1 teaspoon green chrome oxide dispersed into 1 tablespoon avocado oil

1 teaspoon ultramarine blue dispersed into 1 tablespoon avocado oil

Regular lavender essential oil will work, but this variety has been specifically blended to last in cold-process soap.

Note: You may want a pouring buddy for this. If you do ask someone to pour one side of the soap while you pour the other side, make sure they fully suit up for safety, including gloves and goggles.

Safe Soaping!

Wear proper safety gear the whole time.

Work in a well-ventilated space.

No distractions (keep kids and pets away).

MAKE THE SOAP MIXTURE

1. Measure out the water. Take a small pinch of tussah silk and pull it into individual strands. Spread the silk over the surface of the water (it will float). Add the lye to the water (never the other way around), directly over the silk fibers. Heat is essential to help the silk fibers dissolve. Stir gently until all of the lye and most of the fibers dissolve.

If using sodium lactate, add it to the lye-water and stir to combine. Set the mixture aside to cool until it becomes clear. It is normal to have very small strands of silk floating in the lye-water.

2. Melt the palm oil in its original container, mix thoroughly, and measure into a bowl large enough to hold all of the oils and the lye-water with room for mixing. Melt and measure the coconut oil and add it to the bowl. Add the avocado oil, canola oil, green tea seed oil, and olive oil pure.

3. When the oils are between 90° and 100°F (32–38°C) and the lye-water is between 130° and 135°F (54–57°C), add the lye-water to the oils, pouring it over a spatula or the shaft of the stick blender to minimize air bubbles. Tap the stick blender a couple of times against the bottom of the bowl to release any air that may be trapped in the blades. *Do not turn on the stick blender until it is fully immersed.* Stick-blend for 30 seconds, or until very light trace is achieved.

MIX AND POUR

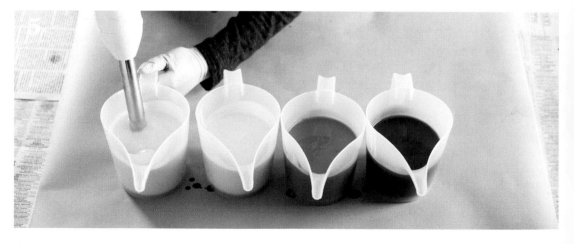

4. Add the essential oil blend, and whisk to combine. Split the batter into four equal containers.

5. Add the following colors to the containers, and stick-blend each for 5 seconds, moving from lightest to darkest to keep from mixing colors.
   » A: 2 teaspoons titanium dioxide dispersion
   » B: 2 teaspoons titanium dioxide dispersion
   » C: 1 teaspoon green chrome oxide dispersion
   » D: 1 teaspoon ultramarine blue dispersion

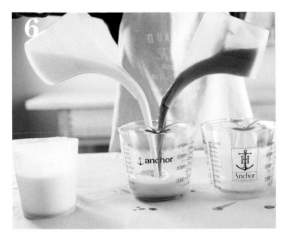

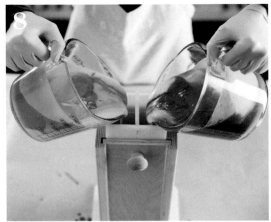

6. Simultaneously pour all of the green soap and one of the white soaps into a larger pouring container, allowing the colors to mix.

7. Simultaneously pour all of the blue soap and the remaining white soap into a larger pouring container, allowing the colors to mix.

8. Simultaneously pour both batches of soap into the mold, with the green mix on one side of the divider, and the blue mix on the other.

9. Pull the center divider straight up and out of the mold.

FINAL STEPS

10. Lightly spritz the top of the soap with 99% rubbing alcohol to help avoid soda ash.

11. Allow the soap to set for at least 48 hours before attempting to unmold. To unmold, first remove the four wing nuts from the front of the mold. Slide off the wooden front, and pull out the entire soap log with the plastic side panels attached. Carefully slide the side panels off the soap; never pull it back and away from the soap, or it will tear.

12. Because the soap wasn't able to breathe inside the mold, allow it to sit in the open for at least 24 hours before attempting to cut it into bars. Once the soap is dry enough, cut into 1-inch bars. Allow the bars to cure in a well-ventilated area for 4 to 6 weeks before using, turning them every few days to ensure that they cure evenly.

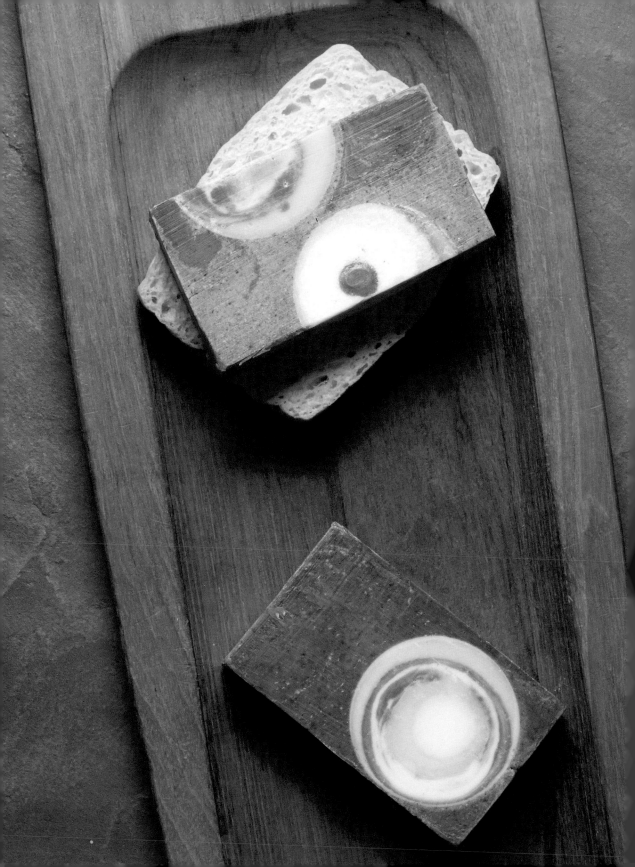

Indigo-Annatto
NEGATIVE-SPACE FUNNEL POUR

Approximately 20 bars

This negative embed technique provides plenty of options for shapes and sizes of embeds, so you are not limited by the type of mold. For this particular soap, a length of simple PVC plumbing pipe was cut into small pieces to create the negative space. The funnel-pour inside the negative space features bright yellow from the annatto infusion, creating a dramatic contrast with the dark blue-gray of the indigo. Indigo shows a much more beautiful blue color when a hot gel phase is achieved (see What Is Gel Phase?, page 32).

STAGE 1
MAKE THE BASE SOAP

Mold and Special Tools

» 5-pound wooden mold with sliding bottom with silicone liner
» 7 pieces 1-inch-diameter PVC pipe, each piece 5 inches long, rubbed inside and out with mineral oil or cyclomethicone
» 7 rubber bands (8" circumference, 1/4" width)
» Heating pad

Lye-Water Amounts

4.7 ounces lye (5% superfat)
11.5 ounces distilled water
1.5 tablespoons indigo powder
1 tablespoon sodium lactate (highly recommended)

Essential Oil Blend

1 ounce lemongrass essential oil
0.5 ounce rosemary essential oil

Oil Amounts

3.5 ounces avocado oil (10%)
8.8 ounces canola oil (25%)
8.8 ounces rice bran oil (25%)
8.8 ounces coconut oil (25%)
5.3 ounces shea butter (15%)

Colorant

1 tablespoon alkanet root powder dispersed into 1 ounce sunflower oil
1 teaspoon titanium dioxide dispersed into 1 tablespoon sunflower oil

Note: Allow yourself two separate days in addition to curing time to create this unique pattern.

Safe Soaping!

Wear proper safety gear the whole time.

Work in a well-ventilated space.

No distractions (keep kids and pets away).

PREPARE THE MOLD

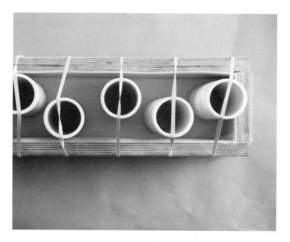

It's important to lubricate the molds with a substance that will not saponify when the raw soap touches it; mineral oil is fine or use cyclomethicone (liquid silicone).

Place the seven lubricated PVC tubes in the silicone-lined mold, spacing them evenly so they are not touching the sides of the mold or each other.

Next, stretch rubber bands around the mold and the PVC tubes. The bands must be tight enough to secure the tubes to the floor of the mold so no soap can seep in.

MAKE THE SOAP MIXTURE

1. Add the lye to the water (never the other way around) and stir gently until all of the lye is dissolved.

2. Add the indigo powder, and whisk in. The powder can sometimes be difficult to combine, but keep stirring until it is all incorporated. If using sodium lactate, add it to the lye-water and stir to combine. Set the mixture aside to cool.

3. In a bowl large enough to hold all the oils and the lye-water solution with room for mixing, measure out the avocado oil, canola oil, and rice bran oil. In a separate container, measure out and melt the coconut oil and shea butter. Once they are completely melted, combine with the other oils.

4. In order to bring out the best color for the indigo powder, the soap must go through a hot gel phase, meaning that the oil temperature needs to be at least 120° to 130°F (49–54°C), and the lye-water around the same. If needed, microwave the entire oil mixture in 15-second bursts to achieve this temperature. Stir the lye-water to incorporate any indigo that may have settled.

Gently pour the lye-water into the oils over a spatula or the shaft of the stick blender to minimize air bubbles. Tap the stick blender a couple of times against the bottom of the bowl to release any air that may be trapped in the blades. *Do not turn on the stick blender until it is fully immersed.* Stick-blend for 20 seconds, or until very thin trace is achieved.

COLOR AND POUR

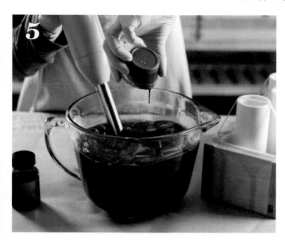

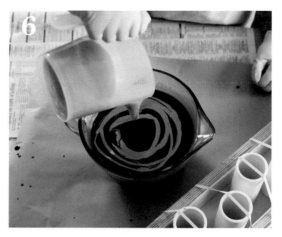

5. Add all of the dispersed alkanet root powder, and the essential oil blend. Stick-blend for about 1 minute.

Split off approximately 12 ounces of batter into an easy-pour container. Add all of the titanium dioxide, and stick-blend for 5 seconds.

6. Pouring from at least 6 inches above the bowl, pour the whitened soap batter into the dark batter in a spiral pattern, using it all.

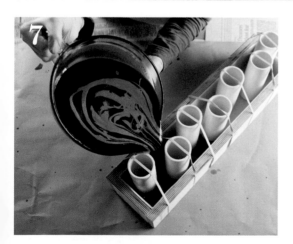

8. Place the mold on a heating pad, and insulate and cover. Leave the heating pad on medium heat for approximately 30 minutes, checking on it often for overheating (signs of this will include cracking, bubbling, or the soap rising). Turn off the heating pad, and leave covered for 24 hours. Do not unmold the soap.

7. Pour the soap batter into one corner of the mold, allowing the batter to fill the mold on its own. If the batter builds up around the tubes instead of flowing, tap the mold gently on the table to settle the soap.

PULL THE TUBES

9. Slowly and gently pull out each PVC tube from the base soap. Do not twist the tube, or you can tear the soap. Use one hand to grasp the tube and pull straight up, while the other hand pushes against the soap to avoid it lifting up. If the columns do not release, allow the soap to set another 24 hours and try again.

STAGE 2:
DO THE FUNNEL POUR

Mold

» 5-pound wooden mold with sliding bottom with silicone liner

Lye-Water Amounts

2.9 ounces lye (5% superfat)

7.3 ounces distilled water

2 teaspoons sodium lactate (optional)

Oil Amounts

5.5 ounces canola oil (25%)

2.2 ounces avocado oil (10%)

5.5 ounces rice bran oil (25%)

5.5 ounces coconut oil (25%)

3.3 ounces shea butter (15%)

Essential Oil Blend

0.7 ounce lemongrass essential oil

0.3 ounce rosemary essential oil

Colorant and Additive Amounts

1 teaspoon titanium dioxide dispersed into 1 tablespoon avocado oil

2 tablespoons annatto infusion*

1 teaspoon black oxide dispersed into 1 tablespoon avocado oil

See pages 48–49 for instructions on infusing herbs.

MAKE THE SOAP MIXTURE

1. Add the lye to the water (never the other way around) and stir gently until all of the lye is dissolved. If using sodium lactate, add it to the lye-water and stir to combine. Set the mixture aside to cool until it becomes clear.

2. In a container large enough to hold all of the oils and lye-water with room for mixing, measure out the canola oil, avocado oil and rice bran oil. In a separate container, measure out and heat the coconut oil and shea butter in 20-second bursts until clear and melted. Add these to the other oils.

3. When the oils and lye-water are between 110° and 120°F (43–49°C), add the lye-water to the oils, pouring it over a spatula or the shaft of the stick blender to minimize air bubbles. Tap the stick blender a couple of times against the bottom of the bowl to release any air that may be trapped in the blades. *Do not turn on the stick blender until it is fully immersed.* Stick-blend for 25 seconds, or until light trace is achieved.

4. Split the soap batter into three equal batches. Add the colorants as follows.

- » Container A: 1 tablespoon titanium dioxide dispersion and one-third of the essential oil blend
- » Container B: All of the annatto infusion and one-third of the essential oil blend
- » Container C: ³/₄ teaspoon black oxide dispersion and one-third of the essential oil blend

5. Whisk all of the containers to incorporate the essential oil and colors.

POUR THE SOAP

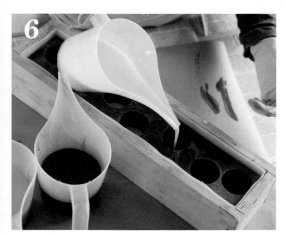 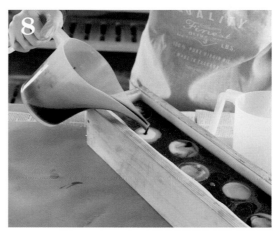

6. Starting with the white soap (Container A), pour the batter into the holes left by the cylinders. From at least 6 inches above the mold, pour a thin, steady stream for a count of 3 into each hole.

7. Repeat step 6 with the orange soap (Container B), pouring directly into the center of the white batter. Pour from high up so that the orange soap breaks through the white soap.

8. Repeat step 6 with the black soap (Container C). Continue the pattern in that order — white, orange, black — until all of the soap is used or the holes are filled.

FINAL STEPS

9. Allow the soap to set for at least 48 hours before attempting to unmold. To remove the sliding bottom, turn the entire mold on its side and pull the bottom out.

10. This recipe uses a different cutting technique to best highlight the design. Cut the log into 3-inch-wide slices. Cut each slice in half horizontally, to expose a cross section of the multicolored circles.

11. Allow the bars to cure in a well-ventilated area for 4 to 6 weeks before using, turning them every few days to ensure that they cure evenly.

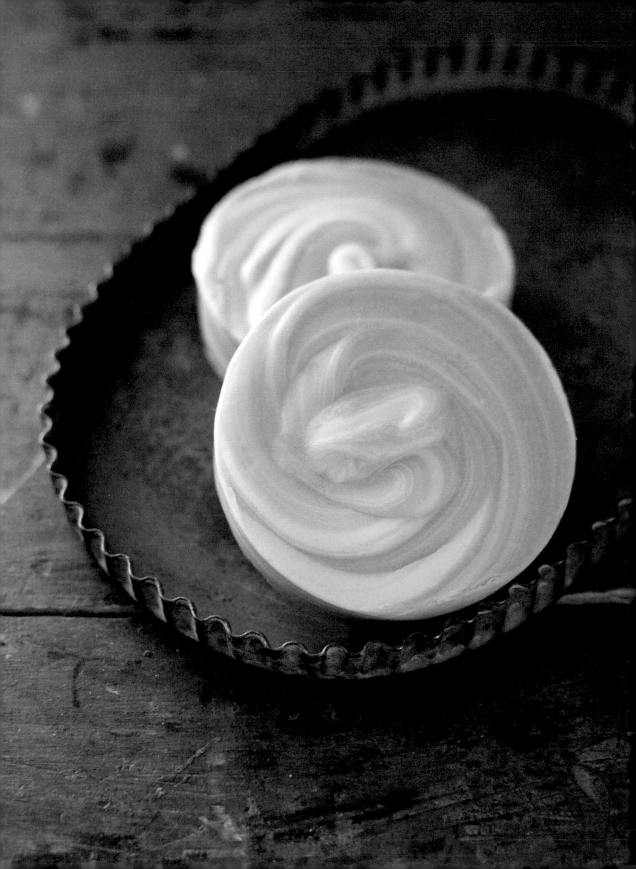

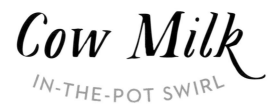

Cow Milk
IN-THE-POT SWIRL

Makes 12 bars

Cow milk contains large quantities of vitamin B_{12} and vitamin D, both of which promote healthy skin. The circular bars from this mold fit perfectly in the hand, and the beautiful spiral-poured swirl adds interest to the bars. The cow milk is added at thin trace to help keep a beautifully neutral color. Burned milk equals brown soap. However, if you neglect to lightly warm the milk, it will cool down the solid oils and result in an accelerated trace.

Mold and Special Tools

» 12-bar round silicone mold placed on a cutting board for easy transportation
» Chopstick or similarly sized swirling tool

Lye-Water Amounts

4.3 ounces lye (5% superfat)
6.9 ounces distilled water
1 tablespoon sodium lactate (optional)

Oil Amounts

5 ounces palm oil (15%)
5 ounces coconut oil (15%)
1.3 ounces avocado oil (4%)
2.6 ounces meadowfoam oil (8%)
2.6 ounces sweet almond oil (8%)
16.5 ounces olive oil pure (50%)

Essential Oil Blend

1 ounce lime essential oil
0.2 ounce basil essential oil
0.5 ounce lavender 40/42 essential oil*

Colorant and Additive Amounts

4 ounces cow milk, lightly warmed to around 90°F (32°C)
1 teaspoon titanium dioxide dispersed into 1 tablespoon avocado oil
1 teaspoon yellow oxide dispersed into 1 tablespoon avocado oil
0.2 ounce orange 10x essential oil
1 teaspoon green chrome oxide dispersed into 1 tablespoon avocado oil

Regular lavender essential oil will work, but this variety has been specifically blended to last in cold-process soap.

Safe Soaping!

Wear proper safety gear the whole time.

Work in a well-ventilated space.

No distractions (keep kids and pets away).

MAKE THE SOAP MIXTURE

1. Add the lye to the water (never the other way around) and stir gently until all of the lye is dissolved. If using sodium lactate, add it to the lye-water and stir to combine. Set the mixture aside to cool until it becomes clear.

2. Melt the palm oil in its original container, mix it thoroughly, and measure into a bowl large enough to hold all of the oils and the lye-water with room for mixing. Melt and measure the coconut oil and add it to the bowl. Add the avocado oil, meadow-foam oil, sweet almond oil, and olive oil pure.

3. When both the oils and the lye-water are between 110° and 120°F (43–49°C), add the lye-water to the oils, pouring it over a spatula or the shaft of the stick blender to minimize air bubbles. Tap the stick blender a couple of times against the bottom of the bowl to release any air that may be trapped in the blades. *Do not turn on the stick blender until it is fully immersed.* Stick-blend for 30 seconds, or until very light trace is achieved.

4. Slowly add the warmed milk to the batter, and stick-blend again for 5 seconds. The soap will be very thin still, but should be uniform in appearance.

COLOR AND SWIRL

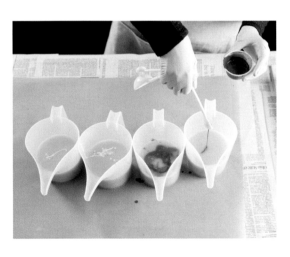

5. Divide the batter equally into four easy-pour containers and add the colorants as follows:
> » Container A: half of the titanium dioxide dispersion
> » Container B: half of the titanium dioxide dispersion
> » Container C: 1 teaspoon yellow oxide dispersion and 0.2 ounce orange 10x essential oil
> » Container D: ½ teaspoon green chrome oxide dispersion

Divide the essential oil blend evenly among the containers, and whisk to combine. Stick-blend each container for only about 2 seconds to blend in the color.

Note: This soap most likely will not gel, but if you are soaping in a hot room, be sure to run a fan over the soap. Gelling the soap will scorch the milk, producing an unpleasant odor and turning the sugars in the milk brown.

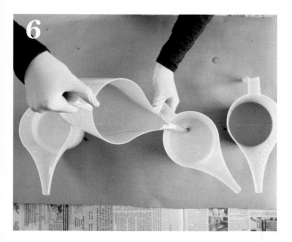

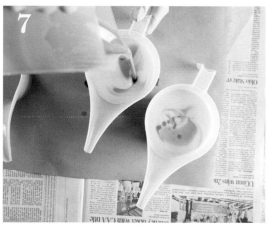

6. Pour half of the yellow batter (Container C) into Container A, pouring from at least 6 inches above the container to allow the yellow to penetrate deep into the white. Pour the other half into Container B.

7. Pour half of the green batter (Container D) into Container A, again pouring from up high so the colors mix. Pour the other half into Container B.

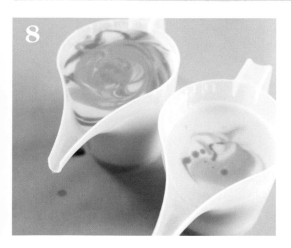

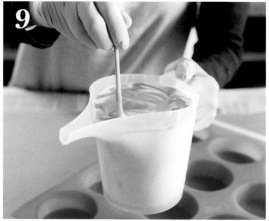

8. When you are finished, you should have two containers holding all the soap batter, with the green and yellow batter equally divided between the two white batches.

9. Using a chopstick, swirl the batter in both containers in a figure eight pattern, just once. Don't over stir! Place the mold on a cutting board so it can easily be moved when full.

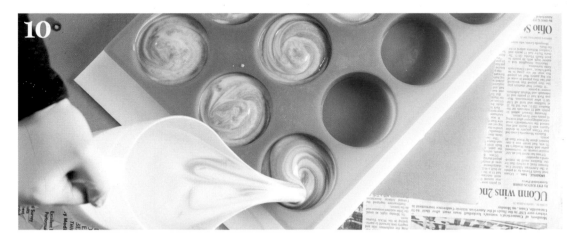

10. Using a spiral motion, pour the batter into each cavity of the mold.

FINAL STEPS

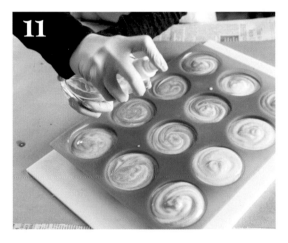

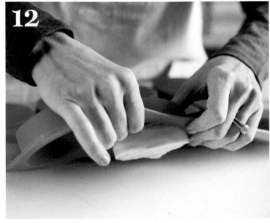

11. Spritz the soaps with 99% rubbing alcohol to help avoid soda ash. Allow the soap to set for 48 to 72 hours before attempting to unmold. A trick for unmolding this type of mold is to place the entire tray in the freezer for 4 to 24 hours, and unmolding the bars while they are frozen to avoid tearing.

12. Once unmolded, allow the soaps to cure in a well-ventilated area for 4 to 6 weeks before using, turning them every few days to ensure that they cure evenly.

Aloe Vera

HANGER SWIRL

Approximately 20 bars

This recipe contains leaves from the aloe vera plant, which the ancient Egyptians called the "Plant of Immortality." Aloe vera has many skin benefits and is used in numerous ways for its soothing and moisturizing properties. Aloe contains choline, which is added to skincare products to help with skin elasticity. This design technique uses a wire hanger to create a fun pattern. Every bar will be unique due to the random spoon-plop technique. Whether you swirl a lot or swirl a little is up to you!

Mold and Special Tools

- » 5-pound wooden mold with sliding bottom with silicone liner
- » Hanger swirling tool (see page 142)
- » 3 large spoons
- » Chopstick or similarly sized swirling tool

Lye-Water Amounts

7.5 ounces lye (5% superfat)

13.1 ounces distilled water

1½ tablespoons sodium lactate (optional)

Oil Amounts

13.7 ounces coconut oil (25%)

5.5 ounces deodorized cocoa butter (10%)

22 ounces olive oil pure (40%)

11 ounces rice bran oil (20%)

2.7 ounces castor oil (5%)

Essential Oil Blend

0.7 ounce cedarwood essential oil

1.8 ounces lavender 40/42 essential oil*

Colorant and Additive Amounts

3 ounces aloe vera leaf, puréed until smooth

2 ounces commercial aloe vera liquid

1 teaspoon titanium dioxide dispersed into 1 tablespoon rice bran oil

1 teaspoon green chrome oxide dispersed into 1 tablespoon rice bran oil

1 teaspoon hydrated chrome green oxide dispersed into 1 tablespoon rice bran oil

Regular lavender essential oil will work, but this variety has been specifically blended to last in cold-process soap.

Safe Soaping!

Wear proper safety gear the whole time.

Work in a well-ventilated space.

No distractions (keep kids and pets away).

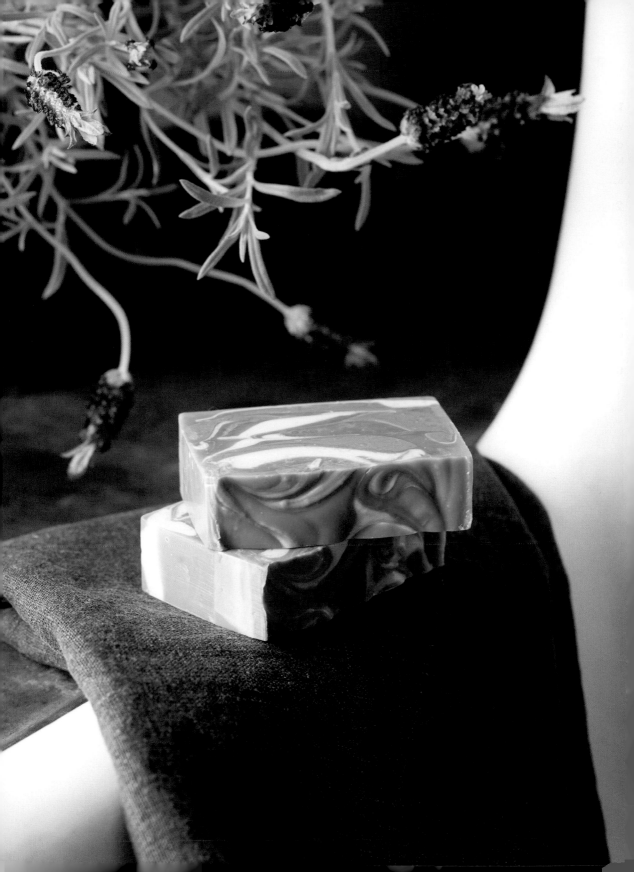

MAKE THE SOAP MIXTURE

1. Add the lye to the water (never the other way around) and stir gently until all of the lye is dissolved. If using sodium lactate, add it to the lye-water and stir to combine. Set the mixture aside to cool until it becomes clear.

2. Melt the coconut oil in its original container, and measure into a bowl large enough to hold all of the oils and the lye-water with room for mixing. Add the cocoa butter to the hot oil. Stir until melted. Measure out olive oil pure, rice bran oil, and castor oil, and add to the hot oil in the large bowl. If the oils become cloudy when the cold oils are added, heat the entire mixture in the microwave until they become clear again. Usually this is around 100°F (38°C).

3. When both the oils and lye-water are between 110° and 120°F (43–49°C), add the lye-water to the oils, pouring it over a spatula or the shaft of the stick blender to minimize air bubbles. Tap the stick blender a couple of times against the bottom of the bowl to release any air that may be trapped in the blades. *Do not turn on the stick blender until it is fully immersed.* Stick-blend for about 15 seconds, or until thin trace is achieved.

4. Add the aloe puree and liquid, and pulse for 5 seconds.

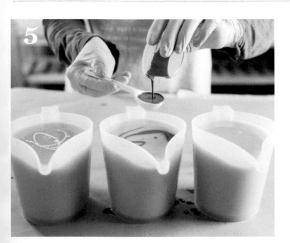

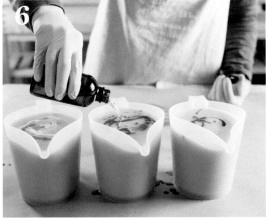

5. Divide the batter equally into three containers. Color the containers as follows:
- » Container A: 1 tablespoon dispersed titanium dioxide
- » Container B: 2 teaspoons dispersed green chrome oxide
- » Container C: 1 tablespoon dispersed hydrated chrome green oxide

6. Divide the essential oil blend evenly among the three containers. Stir the essential oils in well with a whisk, moving from the lightest container to the darkest.

POUR AND SWIRL

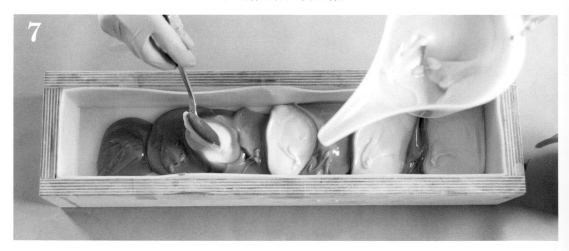

7. Using a large spoon or spatula, plop scoops of soap into the mold one color at a time in a random pattern until all of the batter is used up. Tap the mold on the table after every few passes to release any air bubbles.

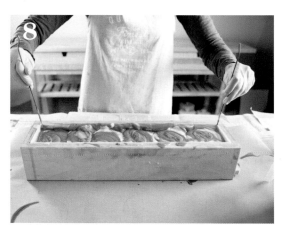

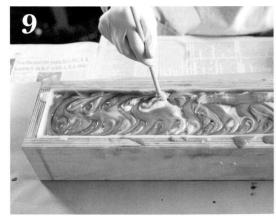

8. Insert the wire swirling tool against one long side of the mold. Slide it across the bottom of the mold approximately 3/8 inch (1 cm), then lift straight up to just below the surface of the soap. Without breaking the surface, move the tool horizontally 3/8 inch (1 cm), then straight to the bottom of the mold. Repeat across the entire mold.

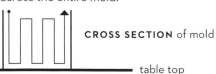

CROSS SECTION of mold

table top

9. Insert the end of a chopstick or skewer about 1/4 inch into the soap batter, starting in a corner. Move the tool in a loop-the-loop pattern across the top.

FINAL STEPS

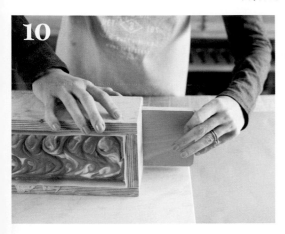

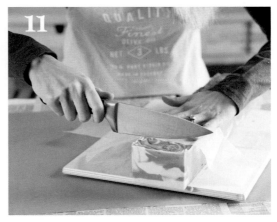

10. Tamp the mold one more time to release any remaining air bubbles. Spritz the top of the soap with 99% rubbing alcohol, then cover it. Allow it to set for 48 hours before attempting to unmold. To remove the sliding bottom, turn the entire mold on its side and pull the bottom out.

11. Once unmolded, cut the soap with a sharp knife in 1-inch slices. Allow the bars to cure in a well-ventilated area for 4 to 6 weeks before using, turning them every few days to ensure that they cure evenly.

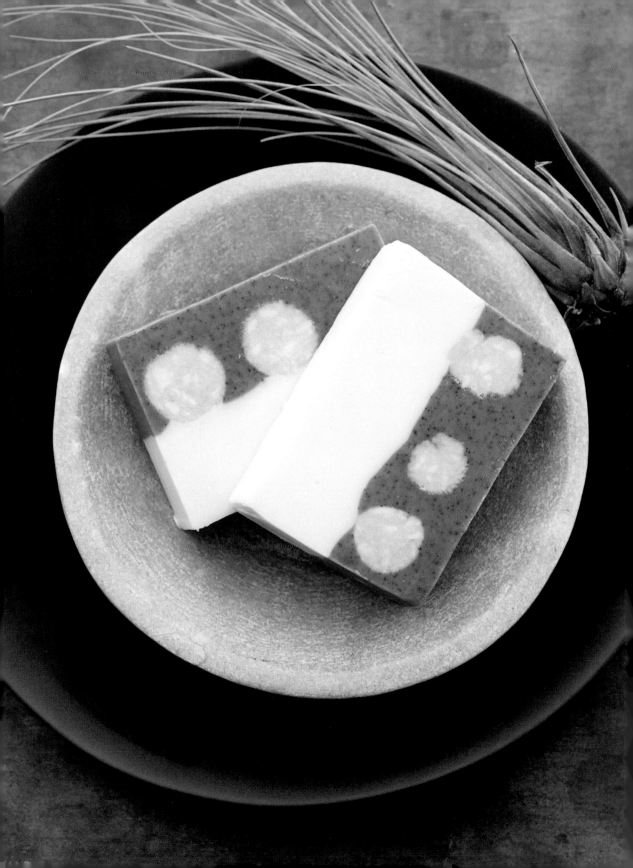

Potato Patch

LAYERED SOAP

Approximately 12 bars

Potatoes are one of the most widely used roots in the world, and are staples in kitchens everywhere. This unique soap, which utilizes real potato puree, is reminiscent of potatoes in a garden. Potatoes are starchy vegetables that some say enhance the skin's natural glow and radiance, and impart moisture to dry skin.

Mold

» 10-inch silicone loaf mold

Lye-Water Amounts

3.9 ounces lye (5% superfat)

7.7 ounces distilled water

1 tablespoon sodium lactate (optional)

Oil Amounts

3.4 ounces palm oil (12%)

7 ounces coconut oil (25%)

1.4 ounces shea butter (5%)

0.8 ounce palm kernel flakes (3%)

14 ounces olive oil pure (50%)

1.4 ounces avocado oil (5%)

Essential Oil Blend

1.1 ounces lavender 40/42 essential oil*

0.4 ounce tea tree essential oil

Colorant and Additive Amounts

8 ounces uncolored, unscented rebatch soap base, grated **

3/4 teaspoon ultramarine pink oxide and 1/4 teaspoon ultramarine violet oxide dispersed into 1 tablespoon avocado oil (purple blend)

1 small potato, peeled

1/2 teaspoon brown oxide dispersed into 1 1/2 teaspoons avocado oil

1 teaspoon ground walnut shells dispersed into 1 tablespoon avocado oil

2 teaspoons titanium dioxide dispersed into 2 tablespoons avocado oil

Regular lavender essential oil will work, but this variety has been specifically blended to last in cold-process soap.

** *You can find grated rebatch in online craft and soaping supply vendors, or you can grate a block of rebatch into smaller pieces to make it easier to melt.*

Note: Allow yourself two separate soaping days — one to create the embeds (plus time to cure) and one for the background soap.

Safe Soaping!

Wear proper safety gear the whole time.

Work in a well-ventilated space.

No distractions (keep kids and pets away).

MAKE THE REBATCH EMBEDS

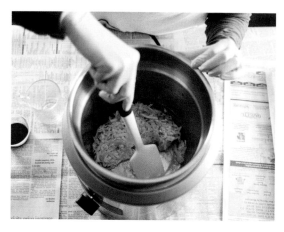
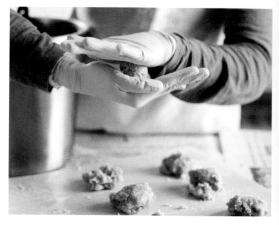

Put the shredded rebatch in a double boiler and melt over high heat for about 15 minutes. Mix in 2 to 4 tablespoons water, depending on the consistency of the soap, until it is the texture of dry mashed potatoes.

Add 1½ teaspoons of the purple blend and mix throughout the rebatch. With gloved hands, roll the rebatch into small "potato balls" while it is still warm and pliable. Set the embeds aside to dry for 24 hours.

PREPARE THE POTATO

Boil the potato in distilled water for about 20 minutes or until it is soft. Combine 2 ounces of the cooked potato and 1 ounce of the potato water, blend until smooth, and set aside to cool.

MAKE THE SOAP MIXTURE

1. Add the lye to the water (never the other way around) and stir gently until all of the lye is dissolved. If using sodium lactate, add it to the lye-water and stir to combine. Set the mixture aside to cool until it becomes clear.

2. Melt the palm oil in its original container, mix thoroughly, and measure into a bowl large enough to hold all of the oils and the lye-water with room for mixing. Melt and measure the coconut oil and add it to the bowl. Add the shea butter and palm kernel flakes to the hot oils, and stir until melted. If needed, heat in microwave in 10-second bursts. Add the olive oil pure and avocado oil.

3. When the oils are between and 95–100°F (35–38°C) and the lye-water is between 130° and 135°F (54–57°C), add the lye-water to the oils. Pour the lye-water over a spatula or the shaft of the stick blender to minimize air bubbles. Tap the stick blender a couple of times against the bottom of the bowl to release any air that may be trapped in the blades. *Do not turn on the stick blender until it is fully immersed.* Stick-blend for 20 seconds, or until very thin trace is achieved.

4. Add the potato-water slurry and the essential oil to the soap. Stick-blend for about 10 seconds, until the potato-water slurry is fully incorporated.

POUR THE BASE

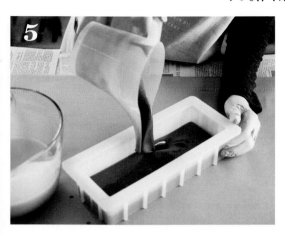

5. Pour about 2 1/2 cups of the soap batter into the first easy-pour container. Add 1/2 teaspoon of the brown oxide dispersion, and all of the walnut shell dispersion. Stick-blend for 5 seconds, then add half of the essential oil. Hand-stir this in, and pour entire mixture into the mold.

ADD THE EMBEDS

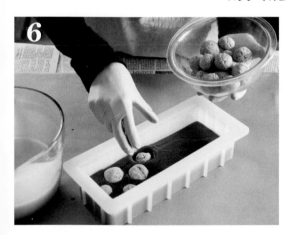

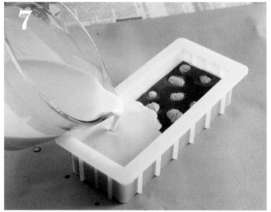

6. Drop the "potato balls" directly into the brown soap in the mold in a random pattern.

7. Add 1 1/2 tablespoons of the titanium dioxide mixture to the remaining batter. Pouring low to the soap, gently pour the white batter over top of the brown layer.

FINAL STEPS

8. Spritz the soap with 99% rubbing alcohol, then cover, and allow the soap to set for at least 48 hours before attempting to unmold.

9. Cut the soap into bars and allow them to cure in a well-ventilated area for 4 to 6 weeks before using, turning them every few days to ensure that they cure evenly.

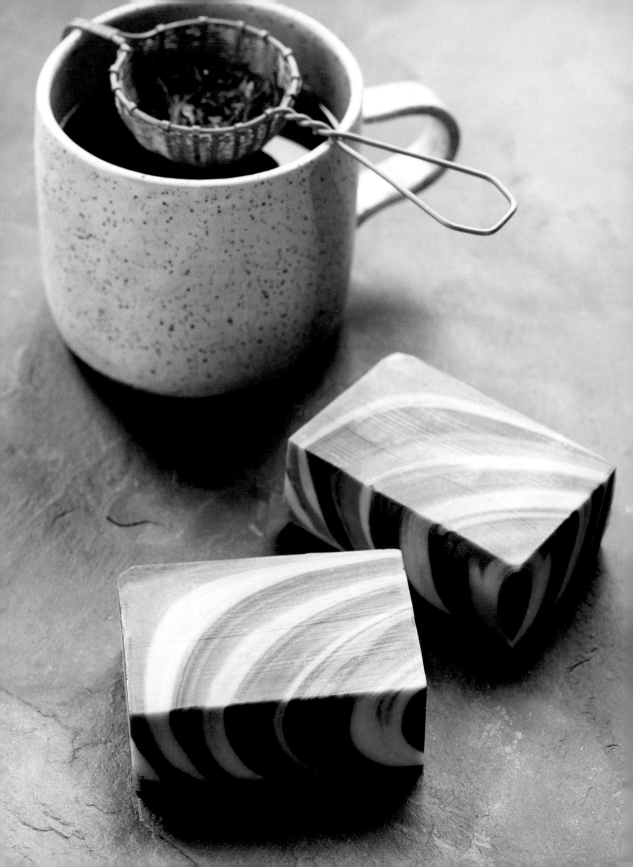

Black Tea
FUNNEL POUR

Makes 9 bars

The rich, invigorating properties of black tea make it a great addition to your soap. Black tea contains tannins, which some studies have shown to improve blood circulation. When lye reacts with black tea, it creates an odd smell and color, but don't worry; the final soap won't be affected. Start with a thin trace to ensure that the pour spreads as far as possible, making beautiful layers.

Mold and Special Tools

- » 9-bar birchwood mold and liner
- » 2 rulers
- » Large (32 ounces) funnel
- » 32-ounce plastic yogurt container or deli container (at least 5 inches tall)

Lye-Water Amounts

- 4.5 ounces lye (5%)
- 5.5 ounces distilled water
- 1 tablespoon sodium lactate (optional)

Oil Amounts

- 8.3 ounces coconut oil (25%)
- 1.7 ounces shea butter (5%)
- 1.7 ounces avocado butter (5%)
- 14.8 ounces olive oil pure (45%)
- 6.6 ounces canola (20%)

Essential Oil Blend

- 1.1 ounces balsam Peru essential oil
- 0.4 ounce bay laurel essential oil

Colorants and Additives

- 1 bag English breakfast or other black tea
- 5.5 ounces distilled water
- 1 teaspoon ultramarine blue dispersed into 1 tablespoon canola oil
- 1 teaspoon titanium dioxide dispersed into 1 tablespoon canola oil
- 1 teaspoon black oxide dispersed into 1 tablespoon canola oil

Safe Soaping!

Wear proper safety gear the whole time.

Work in a well-ventilated space.

No distractions (keep kids and pets away).

PREPARE THE TEA

Add the teabag to 5.5 ounces of boiling distilled water, and steep for 10 minutes. Remove the teabag, and allow the tea to cool to room temperature before soaping.

PREPARE THE MOLD

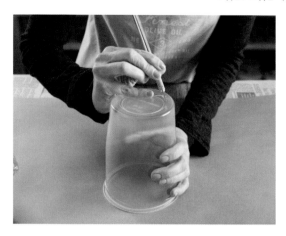

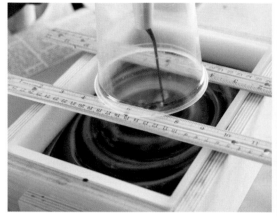

1. Use a sharp blade to cut a hole in the center of the plastic deli cup, large enough to support the funnel, and insert the end of the funnel into the hole. Tape the funnel in place.

2. Place the silicone liner in the mold. Lay the two rulers flat over the center of the mold. Balance the container on the rulers so that the funnel is aimed at the center of the mold.

MAKE THE SOAP MIXTURE

1. Add the lye to the water (never the other way around) and stir gently until all of the lye is dissolved. If using sodium lactate, add it to the lye-water and stir to combine. Set the mixture aside to cool until it becomes clear.

2. Melt and measure the coconut oil into a bowl large enough to hold all the oils and the lye-water solution with room for mixing. Add the shea and avocado butters to the hot coconut oil, and stir until they are melted. If needed, heat in 10-second bursts in the microwave, stirring between bursts, until the butters melt. Add the olive oil pure and canola oil to the hot oils.

3. When both the oils and the lye-water are between 110° and 120°F (43–49°C), add the lye-water to the oils, pouring it over a spatula or the shaft of the stick blender to minimize air bubbles. Tap the stick blender a couple of times against the bottom of the bowl to release any air that may be trapped in the blades. *Do not turn on the stick blender until it is fully immersed.* Stick-blend for 30 seconds, or until thin trace is achieved.

4. Add the black tea and essential oils to the batter. Stick-blend for 5 seconds to combine.

COLOR AND POUR

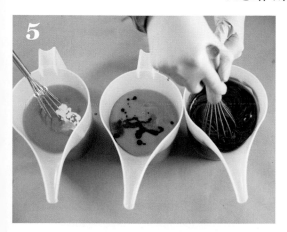

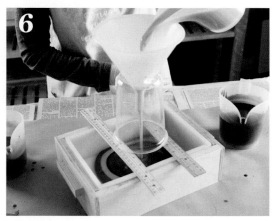

5. Divide the batter equally into three easy-pour containers. Add the following colorants to the containers, and whisk the colors to combine.

» Container A: 2 teaspoons ultramarine blue dispersion

» Container B: All of the titanium dioxide dispersion

» Container C: 1½ teaspoons black oxide dispersion

6. Pour the blue soap batter (Container A) in a slow, steady stream directly into the funnel. Count out loud to 5, and stop pouring. Repeat this process with the white (Container B), then the black batter (Container C), and repeat the pattern — blue, white, black — until all of the batter is gone. If needed, whisk the soap before pouring to help loosen it.

7. Once all of the soap is poured, gently tap and wiggle the mold on the counter to settle the soap. (It has a tendency to pool in the center of the mold under the funnel.)

FINAL STEPS

8. Spritz the soap with 99% rubbing alcohol to help avoid soda ash. Allow the soap to set for 48 to 72 hours before attempting to unmold. If it seems to be sticking to the liner, let it sit for another 24 hours, or place it in the freezer for 4 to 24 hours before trying again.

9. Once unmolded, use a sharp knife to cut the soap into bars. Allow the bars to cure in a well-ventilated area for 4 to 6 weeks before using, turning them every few days to ensure that they cure evenly.

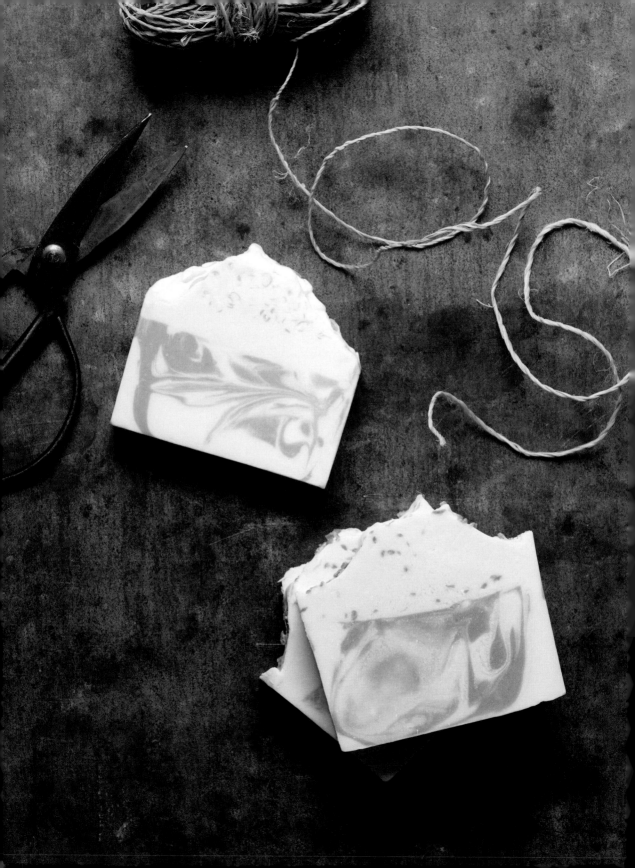

Rosé & Champagne
PEAKS

Makes 9 bars

The beautiful swirls and high toppings of this soap will wow everyone who sees it. Champagne and rosé wine contain antioxidants that promote healthy skin. Egyptian geranium has a roselike scent that matches the look of this soap quite nicely. It is strong, so it can be used at a lower than typical rate and still smell fantastic. The alcohol needs to be reduced and frozen before using it, so plan extra time for that process.

STAGE 1
MAKE THE EMBEDS

Mold and Special Tools
» Small 9-ball silicone mold
» Spare mold to stabilize the 9-ball mold and hold excess soap
» Cheese grater

Lye-Water Amounts
0.7 ounce lye (5% superfat)
1.6 ounces distilled water
¼ teaspoon sodium lactate (highly recommended)

Oil Amounts
0.8 ounce cocoa butter (15%)
2.8 ounces coconut oil (55%)
1.5 ounces olive oil pomace (30%)

Colorants
¼ teaspoon ultramarine pink oxide dispersed into 1 teaspoon olive oil pomace
¼ teaspoon burgundy oxide dispersed into 1 teaspoon olive oil pomace

Essential Oil
0.3 ounce Egyptian geranium

Note: This beautiful design takes two separate soaping days, so plan ahead before making. If you don't care to make the embeds (see photo on page 196), you can skip that step, as shown on the left.

Safe Soaping!
Wear proper safety gear the whole time.

Work in a well-ventilated space.

No distractions (keep kids and pets away).

MAKE THE SOAP MIXTURE

1. Add the lye to the water (never the other way around) and stir gently until all of the lye is dissolved. If using sodium lactate, add it to the lye-water and stir to combine. Set aside until clear.

2. In a bowl large enough to hold all the oils and the lye-water solution with room for mixing, measure out the cocoa butter and coconut oil. Heat in the microwave in 20-second bursts until completely melted. Add the olive oil pomace.

3. When the oils and the lye-water are both between 110° and 120°F (43–49°C), add the lye-water to the oils, pouring it over a spatula or the shaft of the stick blender to minimize air bubbles. Tap the stick blender a couple of times against the bottom of the bowl to release any air that may be trapped in the blades. *Do not turn on the stick blender until it is fully immersed.* Stick-blend for 10 seconds or until thin trace is achieved. Add the essential oil, and whisk to combine.

COLOR AND POUR THE EMBEDS

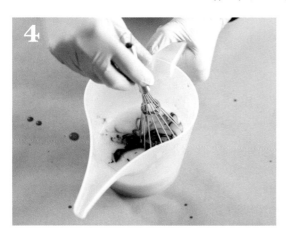

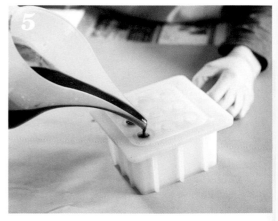

4. Add ¾ teaspoon of the ultramarine pink oxide dispersion and ⅛ teaspoon of the burgundy oxide dispersion, and whisk to combine.

5. Set the 9-ball mold in the spare mold to stabilize it and pour the batter into the openings. Gently tap the mold on the table to release any air pockets. Pour the remaining soap into the spare mold. Allow soap to harden for 24 hours, then pop the soaps out of their molds.

6. Shred the excess soap with the cheese grater, and set aside to use in the final steps.

MAKE THE BASE SOAP

Mold

» 10-inch silicone loaf mold

Lye-Water Amounts

- 5.4 ounces lye (5% superfat)
- 12 ounces rosé wine (4 ounces reduced, per instructions)
- 12 ounces champagne (4 ounces reduced, per instructions)
- 6.2 ounces distilled water
- 1 tablespoon sodium lactate, highly recommended

Oil Amounts

- 1.2 ounces castor oil (3%)
- 3.2 ounces meadowfoam oil (8%)
- 4 ounces sweet almond oil (10%)
- 8 ounces rice bran oil (20%)
- 13.6 ounces olive oil pure (34%)
- 10 ounces coconut oil (25%)

Essential Oil

- 0.9 ounce Egyptian geranium essential oil

Colorant and Additive Amounts

- 2 teaspoons titanium dioxide dispersed into 2 tablespoons sweet almond oil
- 1 teaspoon ultramarine pink oxide dispersed into 1 tablespoon sweet almond oil
- ¼ teaspoon black oxide dispersed into 1 teaspoon sweet almond oil
- Shredded pink soap (made at least 1 day ahead)
- 9 soap ball embeds (made at least 1 day ahead)

PREPARE THE WINE–LYE SOLUTION

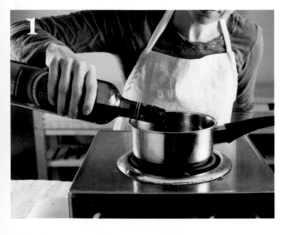

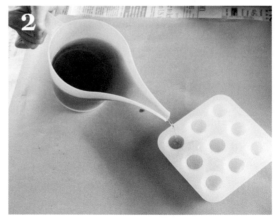

1. Before using the wine and champagne, you must remove as much of the alcohol as possible. Combine 12 ounces of rosé and 12 ounces of champagne in a pot, bring to a boil, then reduce heat to simmer for 15 minutes, stirring constantly. Remove from heat.

2. Once the wine mixture has cooled, measure out 8 ounces, and discard the remainder. Add the 6.2 ounces of distilled water to the wine, pour into an ice cube tray, and freeze completely.

3. Measure the lye into a dry container. Place the ice cubes in a separate heat-safe bowl.

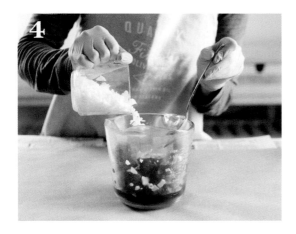

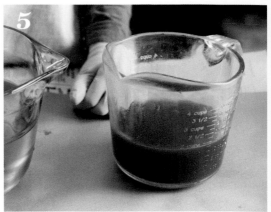

4. Sprinkle or scoop about 1 tablespoon of the lye flakes into the bowl of frozen cubes. Slowly and carefully stir the lye around the cubes, which will begin to melt. After the first spoonful of lye dissolves, add another tablespoon, and stir to combine. Continue this process slowly; it should take about 10 minutes. If you add the lye too fast, the mixture may boil over.

5. Once all of the lye is added and the cubes are melted, add the sodium lactate and stir to combine. Set aside. Note that the solution will remain cloudy instead of clearing as typical lye-water does.

MAKE THE SOAP MIXTURE

1. In a bowl large enough to hold all the oils and the lye solution with room for mixing, measure out the castor oil, meadowfoam oil, sweet almond oil, rice bran oil, and olive oil pure with room for mixing. Heat the coconut oil in its original container, and add the needed amount to the liquid oils.

2. Add the lye solution to the oils, pouring it over a spatula or the shaft of the stick blender to minimize air bubbles. Tap the stick blender a couple of times against the bottom of the bowl to release any air that may be trapped in the blades. *Do not turn on the stick blender until it is fully immersed.* Stick-blend for 20 seconds, or until thin trace is achieved.

3. Divide the soap into three equal parts and whisk in the colorants as follows.

> » Container A: 1 tablespoon titanium dioxide dispersion
> » Container B: 1 tablespoon titanium dioxide dispersion
> » Container C: 1 teaspoon titanium dioxide dispersion, 1 tablespoon ultramarine pink dispersion, $1/16$ teaspoon black oxide dispersion

4. Divide the essential oil equally among the containers. Going from lightest to darkest, stick-blend each container for 2 seconds to combine the essential oil and color. If needed, blend further using a spatula or whisk.

POUR AND SWIRL

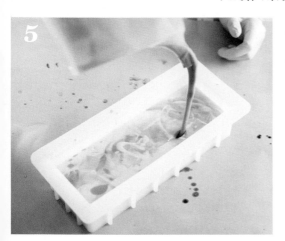

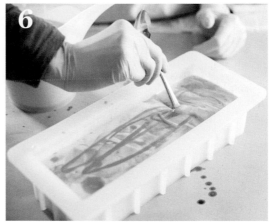

5. Set aside Container A. Begin pouring batter from Containers B and C in random, lengthwise pours from various heights above the mold (from right over the batter to 6 inches or more above). Repeat this process until all of the batter from Containers B and C is used.

6. Insert the handle of the spoon into a corner of the mold at a slight angle. Move the spoon up and down in a figure eight pattern down the length of the mold.

PEAK AND EMBED THE TOP

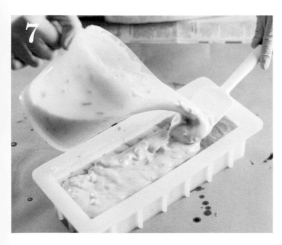

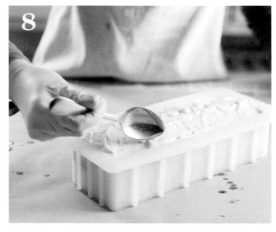

7. Stick-blend the remaining white batter for 5 seconds to bring it to a very thick trace. Once it is thick enough to hold a peak, add ¼ cup of the shredded pink soap to the batter, and stir to incorporate the shreds. Pour this carefully on top of the soap.

8. Using the back of a spoon, pull up the soap from the outer edges to form a peak in the center. If the soap isn't stiff enough to hold its form, let it set a few minutes and try again.

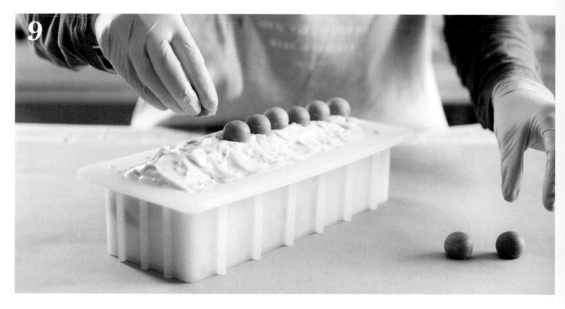

9. Once the top of the soap is sufficiently peaked, insert the round pink embeds. All of them should fit if spaced about ¼ inch apart.

FINAL STEPS

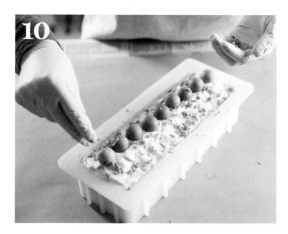

10. Spritz the soap with 99% rubbing alcohol. Sprinkle the entire surface with the remaining pink soap shreds.

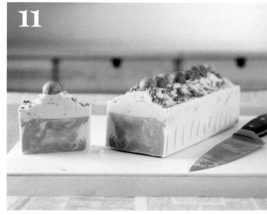

11. Allow the soap to harden for 48 hours before attempting to unmold. To cut this soap, turn it on its side to avoid dragging the soap shreds through the bars. Let bars cure for 4 to 6 weeks before using, turning them every few days to ensure that they cure evenly.

Coconut Milk
SIDEWAYS SWIRL

Approximately 20 bars

This soap has a wonderfully creamy lather, and the sideways hanger swirl and bright colors add lots of visual interest. Thick, rick coconut milk contains lots of vitamins, especially B vitamins, which moisturize skin and promote skin elasticity. It also contains high amounts of sugar, which can heat up soap, so this soap goes into the freezer after it is made. The soap discolors to a light tan if it gets hot and goes through gel phase (see What Is Gel Phase?, page 32). Clear some freezer space before you begin the soaping process.

Mold

- » 5-pound wooden mold with sliding bottom with silicone liner
- » Multi-pour sectioning tool
- » Wire hanger and plastic straws to make swirling tool (see page 142)

Lye-Water Amounts

- 7.6 ounces lye (5% superfat)
- 9 ounces distilled water, frozen into cubes*
- 9.1 ounces coconut milk, frozen into cubes*
- 5 teaspoons sodium lactate (optional)

Oil Amounts

- 11 ounces palm oil (20%)
- 13.2 ounces coconut oil (24%)
- 1.6 ounces avocado butter (3%)
- 3.9 ounces apricot kernel oil (7%)
- 2.8 ounces green tea seed oil (5%)
- 2.8 ounces refined hemp seed oil (5%)
- 19.8 ounces olive oil pure (36%)

Essential Oil Blend

- 2.2 ounces lime essential oil
- 0.3 ounce rosemary essential oil

Colorants

- 2 teaspoons titanium dioxide dispersed into 2 tablespoons avocado oil
- 1 teaspoon ultramarine blue oxide dispersed into 1 tablespoon avocado oil
- 1 teaspoon ultramarine pink oxide dispersed into 1 tablespoon avocado oil
- 1 teaspoon brick red oxide dispersed into 1 tablespoon avocado oil
- 1 teaspoon yellow oxide dispersed into 1 tablespoon avocado oil

*The water and coconut milk can be frozen separately or combined before freezing.

Safe Soaping!

Wear proper safety gear the whole time.

Work in a well-ventilated space.

No distractions (keep kids and pets away).

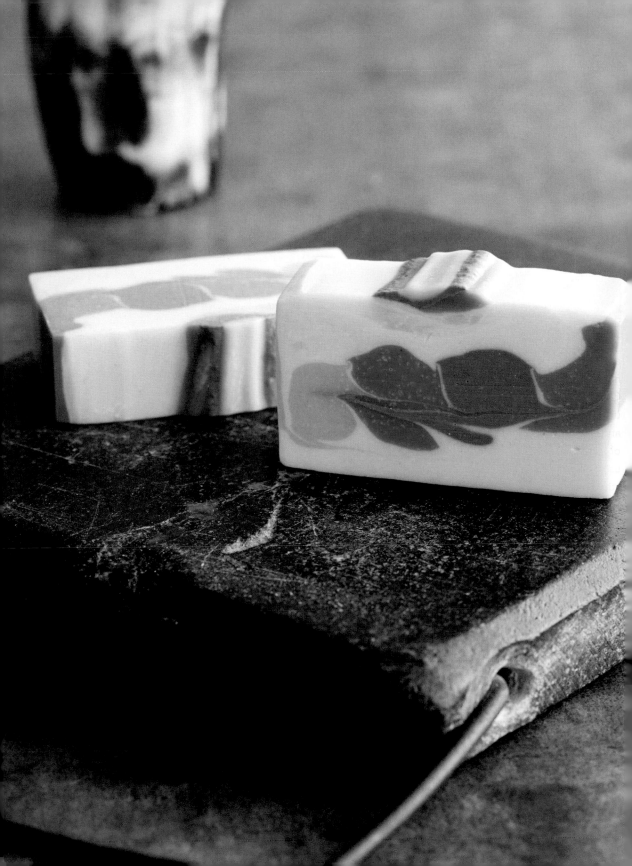

MAKE THE SOAP MIXTURE

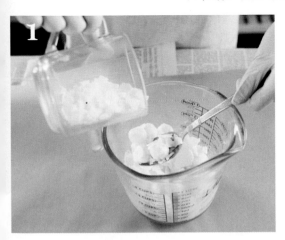

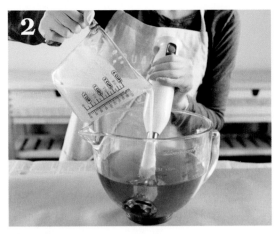

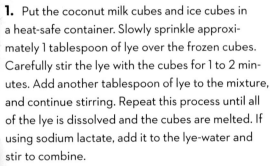

1. Put the coconut milk cubes and ice cubes in a heat-safe container. Slowly sprinkle approximately 1 tablespoon of lye over the frozen cubes. Carefully stir the lye with the cubes for 1 to 2 minutes. Add another tablespoon of lye to the mixture, and continue stirring. Repeat this process until all of the lye is dissolved and the cubes are melted. If using sodium lactate, add it to the lye-water and stir to combine.

The mixture may have an odd smell or slight color to it, which is normal as the lye reacts with the coconut milk. To avoid scorching the milk, keep the lye solution under 100°F (38°C). Because the lye is saponifying the fats in the coconut milk, it is normal for there to be some chunks and texture in the lye-water.

2. Melt the palm oil in its original container, mix it thoroughly, and measure into a bowl large enough to hold all of the oils and the lye-water with room for mixing. Melt and measure the coconut oil and add it to the bowl. Add the avocado butter to the hot oils and stir until melted. If needed, heat the oils further until the butter is completely melted. Add the apricot kernel oil, green tea seed oil, hemp seed oil, and olive oil pure.

Note: When buying canned coconut milk, check the ingredient list. Avoid thickeners such as guar gum or carrageenan and added sugars, as additives can react differently with the lye and speed up trace.

3. When the oils are between 90° and 95°F (32–35°C), add the lye solution to the oils, pouring it over a spatula or the shaft of the stick blender to minimize air bubbles. Tap the stick blender a couple of times against the bottom of the bowl to release any air that may be trapped in the blades. *Do not turn on the stick blender until it is fully immersed.* Stick-blend for 20 seconds, or until very thin trace is achieved.

4. Add all of the essential oil, and whisk to combine.

ADD COLORANTS

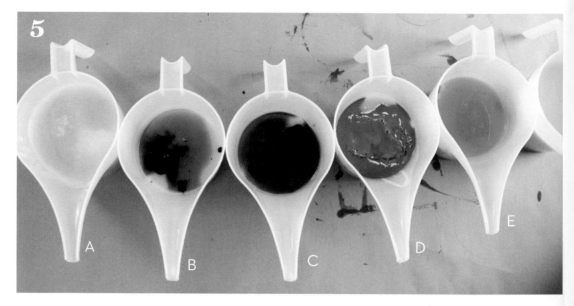

5. Divide the soap into two 20-ounce containers and four 10-ounce containers. Reserve one of the 20-ounce containers until step 10 and add the colorants to the remaining containers as follows.

» Container A (20 ounces): 1½ teaspoons titanium dioxide dispersion
» Container B (10 ounces): ½ teaspoon ultramarine blue oxide
» Container C (10 ounces): 1½ teaspoons ultramarine pink oxide

» Container D (10 ounces): ¼ teaspoon brick red oxide, ½ teaspoon yellow oxide, 1½ teaspoons titanium dioxide
» Container E (10 ounces): ½ teaspoon yellow oxide

Stick-blend each container, moving from lightest to darkest (skip the uncolored one), for about 2 seconds, just enough to blend the color without thickening the trace.

POUR AND SWIRL

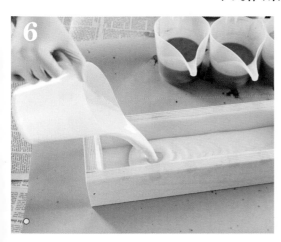

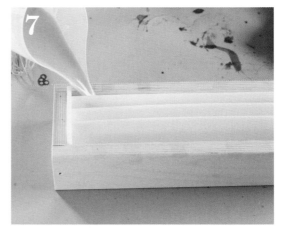

6. Pour the contents of Container A into the silicone-lined mold. Tamp the mold on the table to smooth out the soap. Insert the multi-pour sectioning tool into the mold, creating four equal sections.

7. Pour the yellow oxide batter (Container E) into one of the outside sections, putting the spout as close to the white layer as possible. Pour very slowly and gently to avoid breaking through the bottom layer. Save about 1 tablespoon of the batter for step 12.

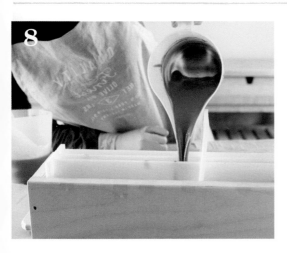

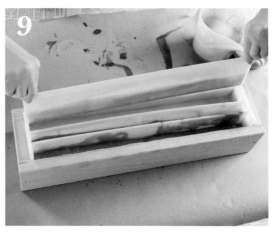

8. Repeat step 7 with the rest of the colors. Pour blue next to the yellow, then orange, then red. It may be necessary to loosen each one before pouring by whisking the batter gently.

9. Once all of the colors are poured, remove the dividers. Slowly pull straight up on each divider until clear of the soap. Don't forget to remove the end pieces.

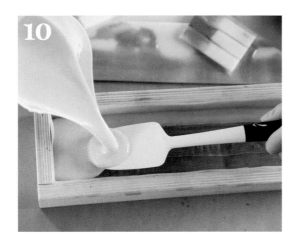

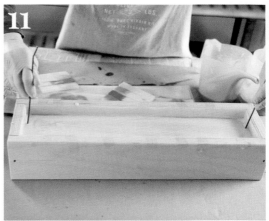

10. Add 1½ teaspoons of titanium dioxide dispersion to the batter set aside in container B. Stick-blend for just a couple of seconds — it needs to be very thin. Pour this layer low and slow over a spatula so you don't break through the colored layers.

11. Insert the wire swirling tool tight along the side of the mold closest to you, right to the bottom. Push along the bottom to the opposite side of the mold. Drag the tool up the wall ½ inch, and pull it straight toward you. Slide it up the wall ½ inch, and push it in a straight line to the other wall again, and repeat once more. Lift the tool straight up the edge of the wall and out of the mold.

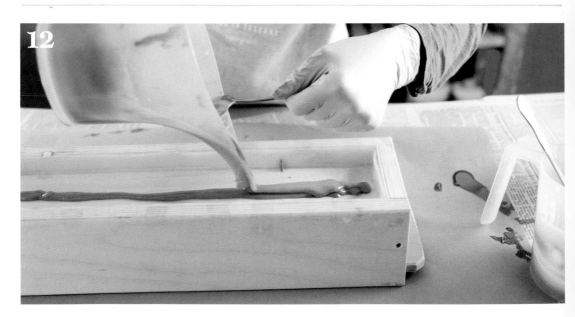

12. Once you are happy with the texture on top, it is time to add more color! Use a spoon to drizzle thin lines of color down the center of the peaks. Layer the colors on top of each other.

FINAL STEPS

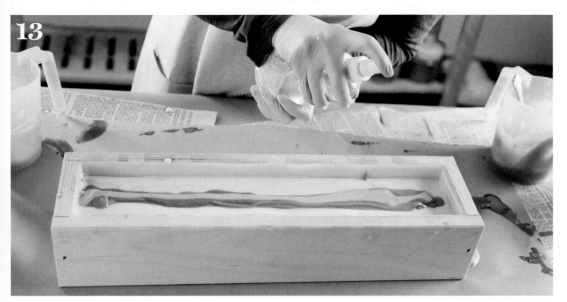

13. Spritz the soap with 99% rubbing alcohol, and place the entire mold in the freezer for 8 to 12 hours. Remove from the freezer, and let stand for 48 hours at room temperature before attempting to unmold.

14. Once unmolded, cut the soap into bars, and allow to cure in a well-ventilated area for 4 to 6 weeks before using, turning them every few days to ensure that they cure evenly.

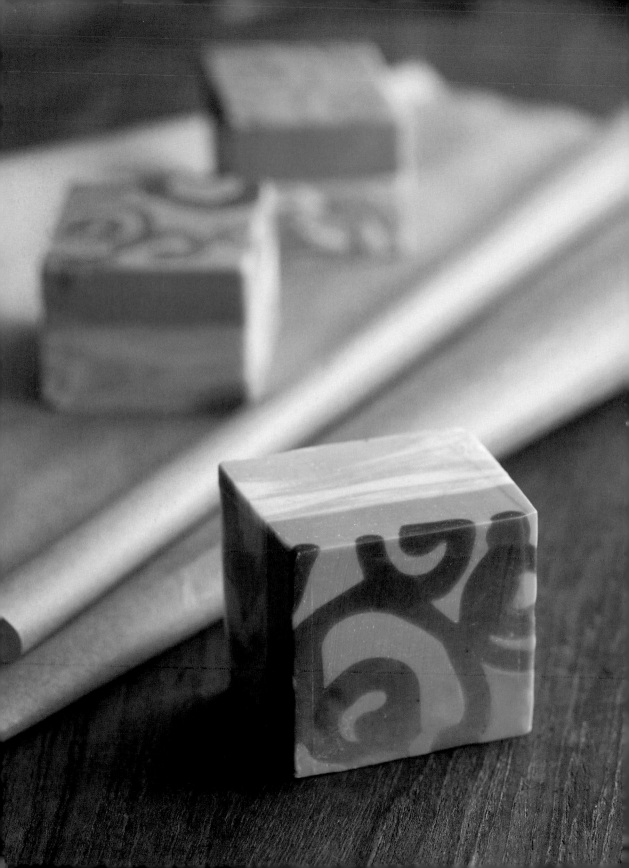

Pale Ale

WITH COCOA POWDER

Approximately 9 bars

This soap is for beer-lovers who would like to actually bathe in beer, or for soap connoisseurs who appreciate the silky-smooth lather that beer adds to the batch. There are numerous options to show off your artistic talents with the cocoa powder swirl — either use this design or create your own pattern for more personalized soaps. To avoid air bubbles on the surface, make sure to pour the first green layer at a thin trace to allow it to flow evenly around the cocoa powder swirls.

STAGE 1
MAKE THE COCOA POWDER SWIRL

Mold and Special Tools

- » 6-inch silicone slab mold
- » Swirl design traced onto a 6- by 6-inch piece of paper
- » Squirt bottle
- » Spare mold for extra soap batter (large enough to hold at least 8 ounces)

Lye-Water Amounts

1 ounce lye (5% superfat)

12 ounces pale ale (reduced per instructions)*

Oil Amounts

1.8 ounces palm oil (25%)

1.8 ounces coconut oil (25%)

0.4 ounce cocoa butter (5%)

0.4 ounce sweet almond oil (5%)

2.8 ounces olive oil pure (40%)

Colorants

2 teaspoons cocoa powder dispersed into 2 teaspoons sweet almond oil

1/4 teaspoon black oxide dispersed into 1 teaspoon sweet almond oil

This makes enough for both parts of the recipe.

Safe Soaping!

Wear proper safety gear the whole time.

Work in a well-ventilated space.

No distractions (keep kids and pets away).

PREPARE THE PALE ALE

Before using the ale, you must remove as much of the alcohol as possible. Bring 12 ounces of pale ale to a boil, then reduce heat and allow it to simmer for 10 minutes, stirring constantly. The amount of liquid that boils off will vary; you need 2.3 ounces of boiled ale for stage 1, and 4.1 ounces of ale for stage 2.

Remove the beer from the heat, and place it in the fridge to cool to between 40° and 55°F (4–13°C). (Beer has less sugar than wine, which creates a very hot reaction with lye; unlike wine, beer doesn't need to be frozen first.)

PREPARE THE MOLD

Create a design on a 6- by 6-inch piece of paper, drawn with dark, thick lines. Lay the paper under the silicone mold (not inside it), taping the edges to keep it from shifting. You should be able to see the lines clearly.

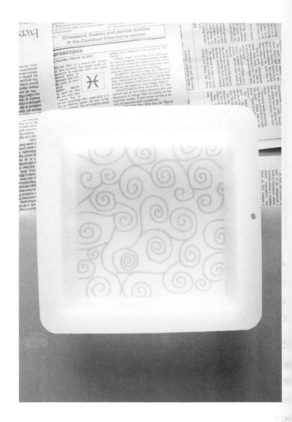

MAKE THE SOAP MIXTURE

1. Add the lye flakes to 2.3 ounces of the cooled pale ale (never the other way around), and stir gently until all of the lye is dissolved. Save the remaining ale for the second part of the recipe.

2. Melt the palm oil in its original container, mix it thoroughly, and measure into a bowl large enough to hold all of the oils and the lye mixture with room for mixing. Melt and measure the coconut oil and add it to the bowl. Add the cocoa butter to the hot oils. Stir until melted. If needed, heat the oils further until the butter and flakes are melted. Add the sweet almond oil and olive oil pure.

3. When the oils are between 95° and 100°F (35–38°C) and the lye mixture is between 125° and 130°F (52–54°C), add the lye mixture to the oils, pouring it over a spatula or the shaft of the stick blender to minimize air bubbles. Tap the stick blender a couple of times against the bottom of the bowl to release any air that may be trapped in the blades. *Do not turn on the stick blender until it is fully immersed.* Stick-blend for 10 seconds, or until very thin trace is achieved.

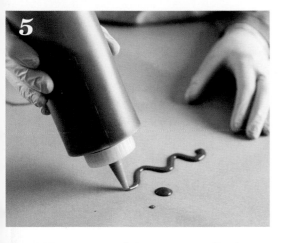

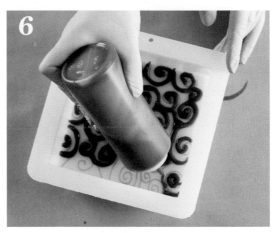

4. Add 3 teaspoons of the cocoa powder dispersion and 1/16 teaspoon of the black oxide dispersion. Stick-blend for 40 seconds, or until thick trace is achieved.

5. Pour the batter into a squirt bottle. Take a piece of plain paper, and create a test swirl. If the design squirts without dripping and holds its shape, it is ready to go. If the design spreads out, or drips as you try to squirt it, allow it to set for another minute and try again.

6. Trace the pattern with the soap. Squeeze lightly, as the design will become muddied if the lines are too thick.

Once the entire pattern is traced, set the mold aside while you make the second part of the soap right away.

7. Because it is hard to stick-blend small amounts of soap, the stage 1 recipe is designed to make more soap than is needed. Pour the excess soap into a spare mold and allow it to cure for 4 to 6 weeks before using.

STAGE 2
MAKE THE MAIN SOAP

Lye-Water Amounts

- 3.4 ounces lye (5% superfat)
- 4.1 ounces distilled water, chilled
- 4.1 ounces previously reduced pale ale, chilled
- 2 teaspoons sodium lactate (optional)

Oil Amounts

- 6.2 ounces palm oil (25%)
- 5 ounces coconut oil (20%)
- 1.3 ounces cocoa butter (5%)
- 1.3 ounces sweet almond oil (5%)
- 3.8 ounces rice bran oil (15%)
- 7.5 ounces olive oil pure (30%)

Colorants

- 2 teaspoons titanium dioxide dispersed into 2 tablespoons sweet almond oil
- 2 teaspoons hydrated chrome green dispersed into 2 tablespoons sweet almond oil

Essential Oil Blend

- 0.5 ounce rosemary
- 0.5 ounce bergamot

MAKE THE SOAP MIXTURE

1. Add the lye slowly to the water and ale (never the other way around) and stir gently until all of the lye is dissolved. If using sodium lactate, add it to the lye solution and stir to combine. Set the mixture aside to cool until it becomes clear.

2. Melt the palm oil in its original container, mix it thoroughly, and measure into a bowl large enough to hold all of the oils and the lye solution with room for mixing. Melt and measure the coconut oil and add it to the bowl. Add the cocoa butter to the hot oils and stir until melted. If needed, heat the oils further until the butter and flakes are melted. Add the sweet almond oil, rice bran oil, and olive oil pure to the hot oils.

3. When both the oils and the lye-water are between 130°and 135°F (54–57°C), add the lye solution to the oils, pouring it over a spatula or the shaft of the stick blender to minimize air bubbles. Tap the stick blender a couple of times against the bottom of the bowl to release any air that may be trapped in the blades. *Do not turn on the stick blender until it is fully immersed.* Stick-blend for 25 seconds, or until thin trace is achieved.

4. Add all of the essential oil blend, and whisk to combine.

COLORING AND POURING

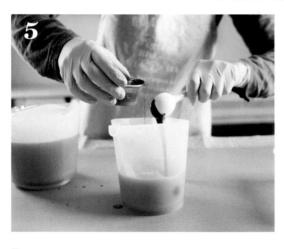

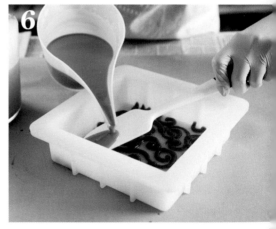

5. Pour off a little more than 1 cup (300ml) of the batter into an easy-pour container. Add to this container 1 teaspoon titanium dioxide dispersion and 2 teaspoons hydrated chrome green dispersion. Stick-blend for 5 seconds to combine the colors.

6. Carefully pour the green batter over a spatula, low and slow, over top of the brown swirls that were made earlier. Gently tap the mold on the counter to bring any bubbles to the surface.

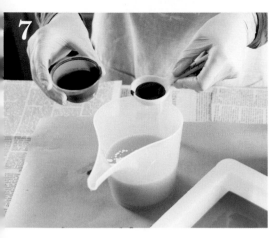

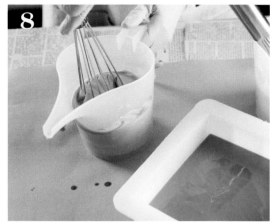

7. Divide the remaining batter into two equal parts and add the colorants as follows:

» Container A: 1 teaspoon titanium dioxide dispersion, 2 teaspoons hydrated chrome green dispersion

» Container B: 1 1/2 tablespoons titanium dioxide dispersion

8. Whisk each container for 3 seconds to incorporate the colors.

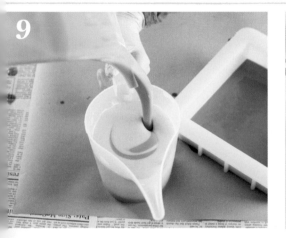

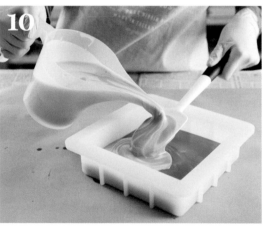

9. Pour the green batter in a spiral pattern into the white batter. Pour from at least 6 inches above to help the green pour all the way to the bottom of the white soap.

10. Pouring over a spatula, carefully pour the swirled green and white soap over the green layer.

FINAL STEPS

11. Spritz the top with 99% rubbing alcohol. Allow the soap to set for at least 48 hours before attempting to unmold.

12. Once unmolded, cut the soap into bars with a sharp knife. Allow them to cure in a well-ventilated area for 4 to 6 weeks before using, turning them every few days to ensure that they cure evenly.

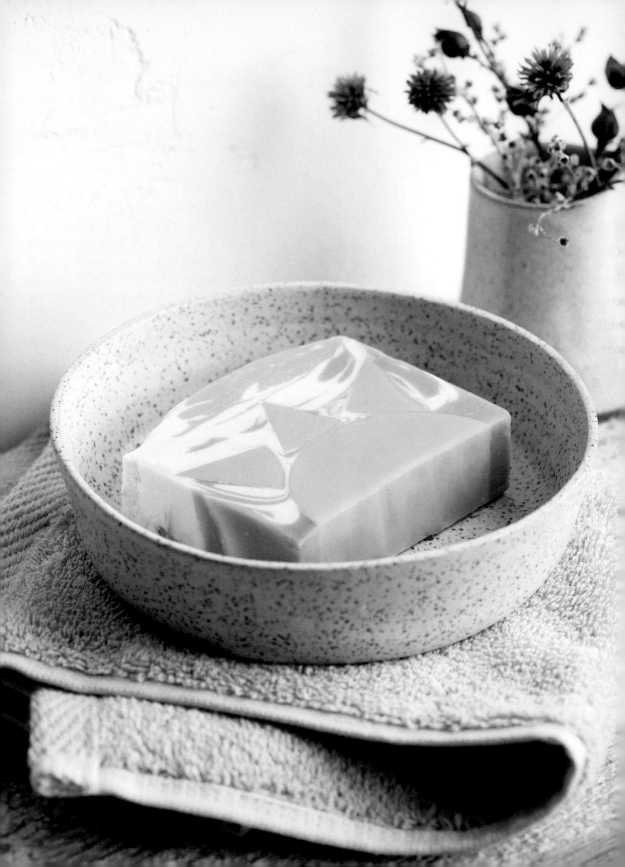

Goat Milk

SUNSET BURST

Approximately 12 bars

Goat milk has long been a favorite ingredient in homemade soaps. It is particularly moisturizing and nourishing to the skin because of the caprylic and capric triglycerides it contains. The protein strands in goat milk are shorter and more readily absorbed by the skin than those in other milks. Goat milk also has naturally occurring lactic acid, as well as vitamins A, D, and B_6.

STAGE 1
CREATE THE EMBEDS

Mold
» 6-cavity half-cylinder silicone mold

Lye-Water Amounts
2.4 ounces lye (5% superfat)
4.6 ounces distilled water
1 1/2 teaspoons sodium lactate (optional)

Oil Amounts
3.9 ounces palm oil (23%)
4.3 ounces coconut oil (25%)
1.7 ounces cocoa butter (10%)
0.9 ounce avocado oil (5%)
6.3 ounces olive oil pomace (37%)

Colorant and Additive Amounts
0.7 ounce goat milk powder dissolved in 1 ounce distilled water, per instructions
2 tablespoons annatto seeds in a sealable teabag

Essential Oil
0.7 ounce orange 10x

Note: This beautiful design requires that the embeds cure for 48 hours before using them in the base soap, so plan ahead.

Safe Soaping!

Wear proper safety gear the whole time.

Work in a well-ventilated space.

No distractions (keep kids and pets away).

PREPARE THE OILS

Melt the palm oil in its original container, mix it thoroughly, and measure into a bowl large enough to hold all of the oils and the lye-water with room for mixing. Melt and measure the coconut oil and add it to the bowl. Add the cocoa butter to the hot oils and stir to melt. Microwave in 10-second bursts if needed. Add the avocado oil and olive oil pomace.

Submerge the sealable teabag with annatto seeds in the oils. Place the oils in a double boiler over medium heat for 2 hours to allow the color to fully leach from the annatto seeds into the oils. Allow the oils to cool to between 100° and 105°F (38–40.5°C) and remove the teabag.

PREPARE THE GOAT MILK

Warm 1 ounce of distilled water to between 90 and 100°F (32–38°C). Add the goat milk powder to the warm water and whisk well to combine. Skip this step if using fresh goat milk.

Note: To help avoid scorching, this recipe incorporates the goat milk by using a concentrated solution of powdered goat milk. This allows more milk to be added without having to add it directly to the lye. The concentrate is added at trace, when the lye is already reacting with the oils and is becoming less active. To use fresh goat milk, see step 1 for instructions.

MAKE THE SOAP MIXTURE

1. Add the lye to the distilled water (never the other way around) and stir gently until all of the lye is dissolved. If using sodium lactate, add it to the lye-water and stir to combine.
TO USE FRESH GOAT MILK, freeze 5.6 ounces of milk into cubes. Sprinkle the lye directly over the frozen cubes, and stir until all of the lye is dissolved. Do not add any distilled water. Continue soaping as normal, but skip adding milk in step 3.

2. When both the oils and the lye-water are between 100° and 105°F (38–40.5°C), add the lye-water to the oils, pouring it over a spatula or the shaft of the stick blender to minimize air bubbles. Tap the stick blender a couple of times against the bottom of the bowl to release any air that may be trapped in the blades. *Do not turn on the stick blender until it is fully immersed.* Stick-blend for 20 seconds, or until thin trace is achieved.

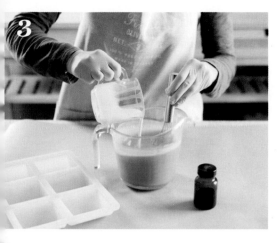

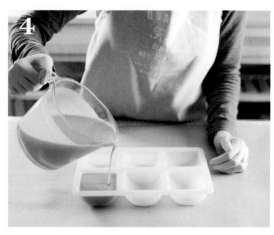

3. Add all of the goat milk and the essential oil to the batter, and whisk to combine. If using fresh goat milk, add only the essential oil.

4. Fill each cavity of the mold to the brim. Spritz with 99% rubbing alcohol and let set for 48 hours before attempting to unmold.

CUT THE EMBEDS

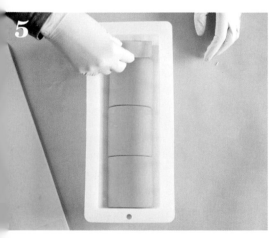

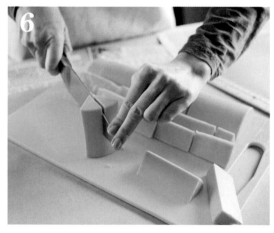

5. Center three embeds flat-side down in the mold. There will be a 1-inch space left. Take a fourth embed, and cut a 1-inch-wide slice off the end. Place the small slice in the mold to be sure it fits.

6. Now there should be two whole embeds and one 2-inch-wide piece. Cut these into lengthwise quarters, so that each embed creates four long, skinny triangles.

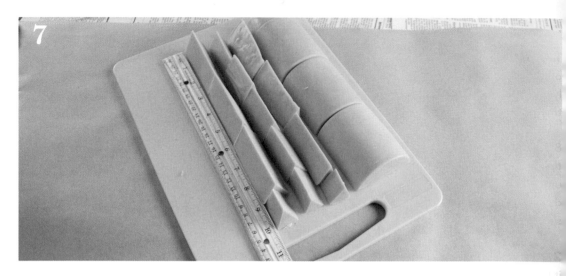

7. Arrange the triangle soaps in three lines next to the half-circle soaps out of the mold to ensure they will fit perfectly. Cut the triangles as needed to make three complete rows of "rays." Leaving them lined up in the correct rows makes it easier to place them when pouring.

STAGE 2
MAKE THE BACKGROUND SOAP

Mold
10-inch silicone loaf mold

Lye-Water Amounts
3.4 ounces lye (5% superfat)

6.3 ounces distilled water

2 teaspoons sodium lactate (optional)

Oil Amounts
3.8 ounces palm oil (15%)

6.3 ounces coconut oil (25%)

1.3 ounces sweet almond oil (5%)

6.3 ounces rice bran oil (25%)

7.5 ounces olive oil pure (30%)

Essential Oil Blend
0.5 ounce bergamot

0.5 ounce lavender 40/42*

Colorant and Additive Amounts
1 ounce goat milk powder dissolved in 2 ounces distilled water, per instructions

2 teaspoons titanium dioxide dispersed into 2 table-spoons sweet almond oil

3 teaspoons ultramarine pink oxide dispersed into 3 table-spoons sweet almond oil

* Regular lavender essential oil will work, but this variety has been specifically blended to last in cold-process soap.

PREPARE THE GOAT MILK

Warm 2 ounces of distilled water to between 90° and 100°F (32–37°C). Add the goat milk powder to the warm water, and whisk well to combine. Skip this step if using fresh goat milk.

MAKE THE SOAP MIXTURE

1. Add the lye to the distilled water (never the other way around) and stir gently until all of the lye is dissolved. If using sodium lactate, add it to the lye-water and stir to combine.

TO USE FRESH GOAT MILK, freeze 8.3 ounces of milk into cubes. In step 1, sprinkle the lye directly over the frozen cubes, and stir until all of the lye is dissolved. Do not add any distilled water. Continue soaping as normal, but skip adding milk in step 4.

2. Melt the palm oil in its original container, mix it thoroughly, and measure into a bowl large enough to hold all of the oils and the lye-water with room for mixing. Melt and measure the coconut oil and add it to the bowl. Add the sweet almond oil, rice bran oil, and olive oil pure.

3. When both the oils and the lye-water are between 95° and 100°F (35–38°C), add the lye-water to the oils, pouring it over a spatula or the shaft of the stick blender to minimize air bubbles. Tap the stick blender a couple of times against the bottom of the bowl to release any air that may be trapped in the blades. *Do not turn on the stick blender until it is fully immersed.* Stick-blend for 20 seconds, or until thin trace is achieved.

COLOR AND POUR

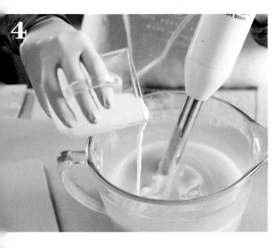

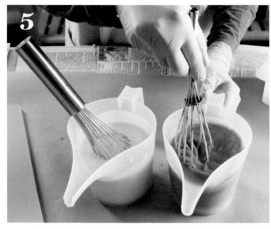

4. Add the goat milk and the essential oil to the soap batter. Whisk to combine. If using fresh goat milk, whisk in the essential oil only.

5. Divide the soap in half and add the colorants as follows.

>> Container A: 1 teaspoon titanium dioxide dispersion

>> Container B: 1 teaspoon ultramarine pink oxide dispersion

CREATE THE SUNBURSTS

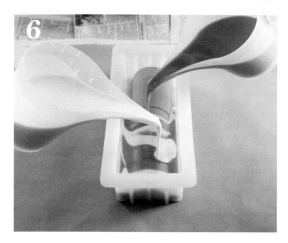

6. Pour random lines of pink and white batter across the round embeds until the batter is almost even with the top of the embeds.

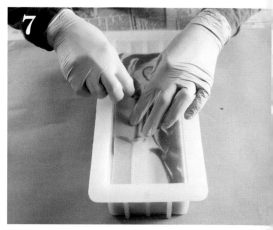

7. Lay the "rays" from the first row of embeds (stage 1, step 7) along one side of the soap. Insert the embeds with the base of the triangle touching, or almost touching the round embeds. Don't let the embed touch the walls of the mold, or the final soap may split.

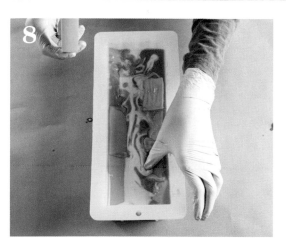

8. Repeat step 7 on the opposite side of the soap.

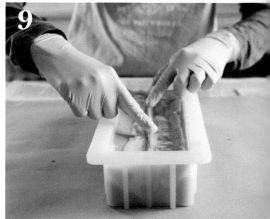

9. Insert the final row of embeds down the center of the soap.

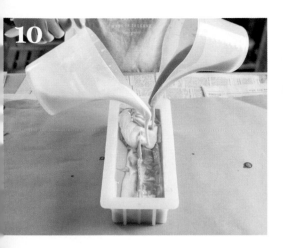

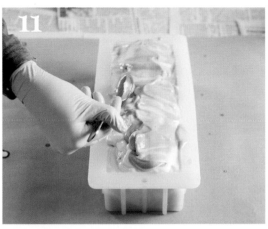

10. Simultaneously pour pink and white batter across the embers until you reach the top edge of the mold.

11. Stick-blend the remaining batter for 5 to 10 seconds, or until very thick trace is achieved. Spoon the batter onto the soap, raising it above the edges of the mold. Use the back of a spoon to smooth and shape the soap into a round peak.

FINAL STEPS

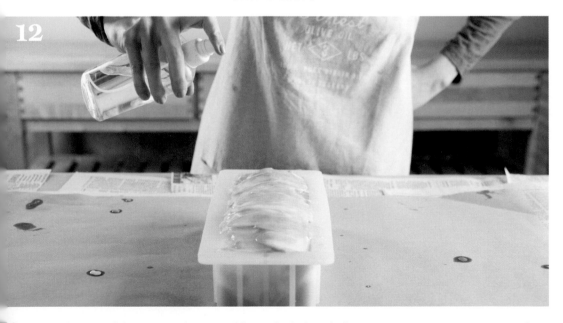

12. Spritz the top of the soap with 99% rubbing alcohol, and allow it to set at room temperature for at least 48 hours before attempting to unmold. Cut into bars, and allow them to cure in a well-ventilated area for 4 to 6 weeks before using, turning them every few days to ensure that they cure evenly.

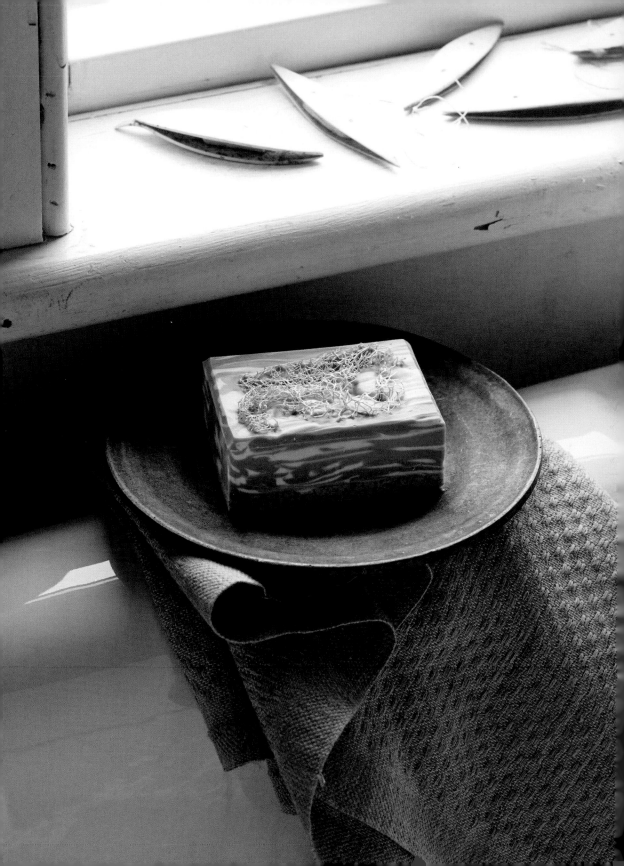

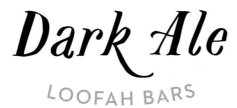

Dark Ale
LOOFAH BARS

Makes 9 bars

This bold, beautiful soap is sure to be a favorite with both men and women. The fresh scent of spearmint and patchouli is perfectly blended so that even those with an aversion to patchouli will love it. The dark ale enhances the lather, while the walnut shell layer on the bottom and the loofah on top create an exfoliating bar. The beer needs to be prepared ahead of time, so plan an extra day when you make this recipe.

Mold
» 9-bar birchwood mold with silicone liner
» 3 squirt bottles

Lye-Water Amounts
4.5 ounces lye (5% superfat)

5.4 ounces distilled water, frozen in ice cubes

10 ounces dark ale (5.4 ounces reduced, per instructions)

1 tablespoon sodium lactate (optional)

Oil Amounts
1 ounce tamanu oil (3%)

1.7 ounces green tea seed oil (5%)

7.9 ounces rice bran oil (24%)

13.2 ounces olive oil pure (40%)

8.3 ounces coconut oil (25%)

1 ounce shea butter (3%)

Essential Oil Blend
0.7 ounce spearmint essential oil

0.8 ounce patchouli essential oil

Colorant and Additive Amounts
9 loofah slices, 1 1/2 by 2 inches across and 1/2 inch thick*

2 teaspoons titanium dioxide dispersed into 2 tablespoons green tea seed oil

2 teaspoons walnut shells

1 teaspoon hydrated chrome green dispersed into 1 tablespoon green tea seed oil

1 teaspoon ultramarine blue dispersed into 1 tablespoon green tea seed oil

*Loofah is a natural product, so the number of slices per piece will vary, but two loofah sponges should be enough.

Safe Soaping!

Wear proper safety gear the whole time.

Work in a well-ventilated space.

No distractions (keep kids and pets away).

PREPARE THE ALE

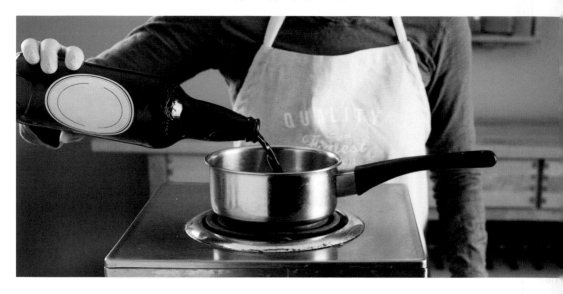

Before using ale in soap, you must remove as much of the alcohol as possible. Bring the ale to a boil, then reduce heat and simmer for 10 minutes, stirring constantly. After the ale cools, measure out 5.4 ounces and freeze it into cubes.

PREPARE THE LOOFAH

If your loofah is flat instead of round, simply dunk the loofah in cold water to re-inflate and let fully dry before using in your soap. Although the divider set is not used in molding this soap, it will serve as a useful tool in figuring out the best layout for the loofah pieces, to get the most striking effect. Before beginning, put the divider set inside the silicone liner. Using a permanent marker, make a small mark on the top edge of the silicone liner where the edges of the dividers hit the walls. The marker can be easily removed with 99% rubbing alcohol when the project is finished.

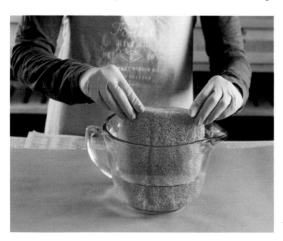 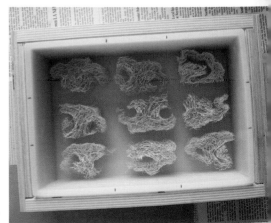

MAKE THE SOAP MIXTURE

1. Measure out the needed amount of dark ale cubes and distilled water cubes. Sprinkle about a tablespoon of lye over the cubes, and stir gently. The lye will begin to melt the cubes. Stir for about a minute, then add another tablespoon of lye. Repeat the process, adding small amounts of lye and stirring, until all the lye has been added. Keep stirring the mixture until all of the lye chunks are dissolved.

2. If using sodium lactate, add it to the lye mixture and stir to combine. Set the mixture aside to cool.

3. In a bowl large enough to hold all the oils and the lye mixture with room for mixing, measure out the tamanu oil, green tea seed oil, rice bran oil, and olive oil pure. In a separate container, heat the coconut oil until liquid, and pour the hot oil over the shea butter. Stir this until the shea butter melts. Add the hot oil mixture to the liquid oils.

4. When both the oils and the lye mixture are between 110° and 120°F (43–49°C), strain the lye mixture as you add it to the oils, pouring it over a spatula or the shaft of the stick blender to minimize air bubbles. Tap the stick blender a couple of times against the bottom of the bowl to release any air that may be trapped in the blades. *Do not turn on the stick blender until it is fully immersed.* Stick-blend for 10 seconds, or until thin trace is achieved.

MIX AND POUR

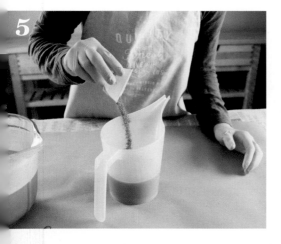

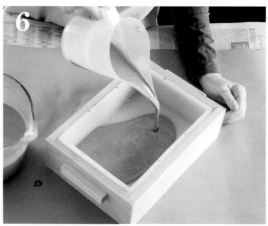

5. Add 1 tablespoon of the titanium dioxide dispersion and all of the essential oil blend. Whisk to combine. Pour off about 1 cup (300ml) of the batter into a small container. Add the walnut shells to this batch and stick-blend for 15 seconds.

6. Pour all of the thickened batter into the bottom of the silicone-lined mold.

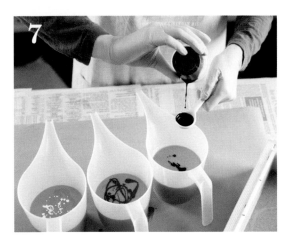

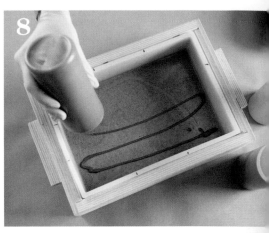

7. Divide the remaining batter into three equal containers. Add the colorants to each container as follows, stick-blending in 2-second bursts to mix.

> » Container A: remaining 1 tablespoon titanium dioxide dispersion
> » Container B: 2 teaspoons hydrated green chrome dispersion
> » Container C: 2 teaspoons ultramarine blue dispersion

8. Pour each container of soap into its own squirt bottle. Gently squirt long lines of each color over the brown layer of soap; squirt low to the soap to avoid breaking through the layer. Continue squirting alternating colors of soap across the surface until all of the batter is used.

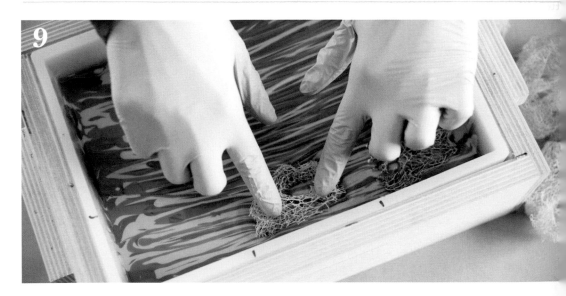

9. Carefully squish each loofah into the soap, being mindful to stay between each of the markings, and leaving just about a ¼ inch of loofah above the surface of the soap.

FINAL STEPS

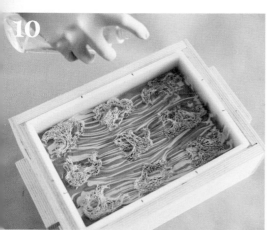

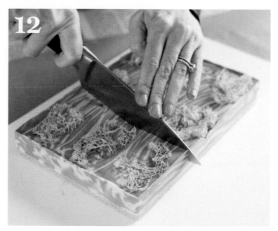

10. Spritz the surface of the soap with 99% rubbing alcohol to help prevent soda ash. This is a fairly soft recipe, so do not attempt to unmold it for 48 to 72 hours.

11. Before unmolding, use a knife to score the soap along the marks made previously. If the soap is sticking to the silicone liner when attempting to unmold, let it set another day.

12. Cut the soap into bars along the scoring lines. Allow the bars to cure in a well-ventilated area for 4 to 6 weeks before using, turning them every few days to ensure that they cure evenly.

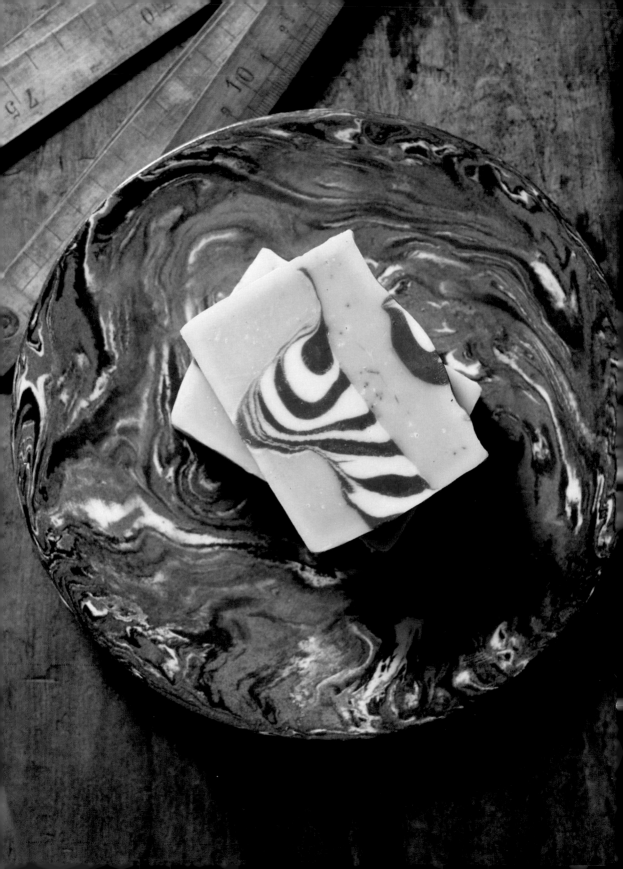

Dandelion

ZEBRA STRIPES

Approximately 8 bars

Dandelions are not just a weed; the nourishing greens have long been used to treat a variety of ailments. The petals add a very soft, mild texture to the bars as well as giving a burst of color that really makes the stripes pop. The awesome zebra stripe technique was first created by Vinvela Ebony from Dandelion Seifee.

Mold and Special Tools

» 2-pound wooden mold with silicone liner
» 1 manila folder, cut to width of the mold, and 5 inches tall
» Chopstick or similarly sized swirling tool

Oil Amounts

2 ounces apricot kernel oil (8%)
3.5 ounces rice bran oil (14%)
3.8 ounces sunflower oil (15%)
9.5 ounces olive oil pure (38%)
6.3 ounces coconut oil (25%)

See pages 48–49 for how to make infused oils.

Lye-Water Amounts

3.4 ounces lye (5% superfat)
8.3 ounces dandelion infusion (10 ounces distilled water infused with 0.5 ounce whole dandelions)
2 teaspoons sodium lactate (optional)

Essential Oil Blend

0.4 ounce peppermint 2nd distilled essential oil
0.6 ounce lime essential oil

Colorant and Additive Amounts

1 teaspoon annatto seeds infused in 1 ounce sunflower oil*
2 heaping tablespoons dandelion petals
1 teaspoon titanium dioxide dispersed into 1 tablespoon sunflower oil
1 teaspoon ultramarine blue oxide dispersed into 1 tablespoon sunflower oil

Note: Pick dandelions from a spot that has not been sprayed with chemicals, and rinse them well before using them in the soap.

Safe Soaping!

Wear proper safety gear the whole time.

Work in a well-ventilated space.

No distractions (keep kids and pets away).

PREPARE THE DANDELION INFUSION

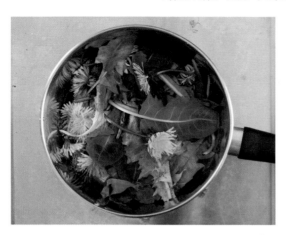

Combine ½ ounce whole dandelions (stems, leaves, and petals) with 10 ounces distilled water in a pot and simmer over medium heat for 15 minutes, or until the water takes on a yellow tint. Strain the dandelions out of the water, and weigh out 8.3 ounces dandelion water. Set aside to cool to room temperature.

MAKE THE SOAP MIXTURE

1. Slowly add the lye to the cooled dandelion infusion (never the other way around), and stir until all of the lye is dissolved. The lye will turn the water a bright orange/yellow color. If using sodium lactate, add it to the lye-water and stir to combine. Set the mixture aside to cool.

2. In a bowl large enough to hold all the oils and the lye-water solution with room for mixing, measure out the apricot kernel oil, rice bran oil, sunflower oil, and olive oil pure. Microwave the coconut oil in 30-second bursts until melted, and combine with the other oils.

3. When the oils and the lye-water are between 110° and 120°F (43–49°C), add the lye-water to the oils, pouring it over a spatula or the shaft of the stick blender to minimize air bubbles. Tap the stick blender a couple of times against the bottom of the bowl to release any air that may be trapped in the blades. *Do not turn on the stick blender until it is fully immersed.* Stick-blend for 25 seconds, or until very thin trace is achieved.

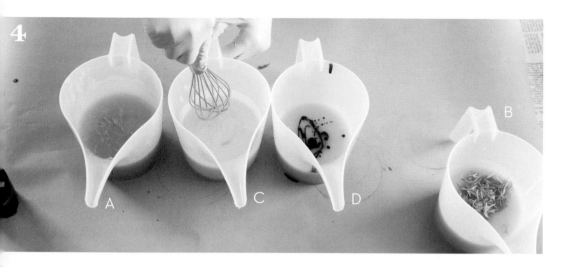

4. Divide the batter into four equal parts and add the colorants and additives as follows.

» Container A: 1 tablespoon annatto infusion, 1 tablespoon dandelion petals, one-fourth of the essential oil

» Container B: 1 tablespoon annatto infusion, 1 tablespoon dandelion petals, one-fourth of the essential oil

» Container C: 2 teaspoons titanium dioxide dispersion, one-fourth of the essential oil

» Container D: 1 1/2 teaspoons ultramarine blue dispersion, one-fourth of the essential oil

POUR, STRIPE, AND SWIRL

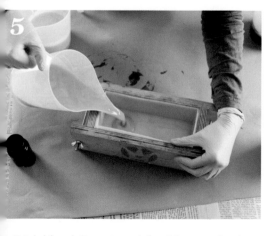

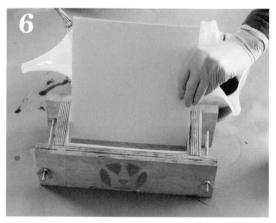

5. Stick-blend Container A for 20 seconds, then pour the batter into the mold. Whisk the remaining colors so as not to accelerate trace.

6. Angle the manila folder into the bottom layer of soap. You want to just touch the first layer of soap without pushing into it.

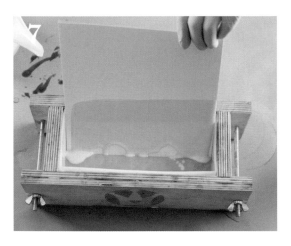

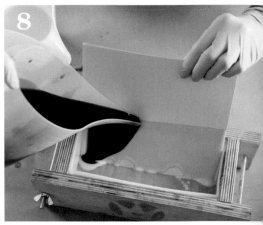

7. Pour a strip of white batter (Container C) across the manila folder, allowing it to run down the paper and across the first layer of soap.

8. Without moving the folder from its original position, pour a strip of blue batter (Container D) across the folder, allowing it to run down the paper and across the white layer.

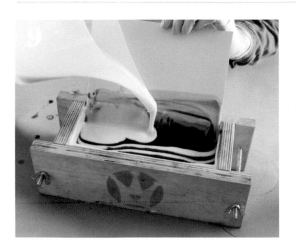

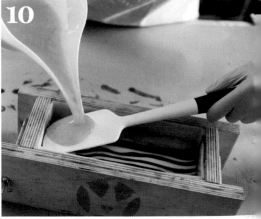

9. Repeat steps 7 and 8, making five passes of each color before removing the folder. You should have about ¼ cup of soap remaining in each container.

10. Whisk the remaining container of yellow soap (Container B) to loosen it. Pouring low and slow over the back of a spatula, cover the blue and white layers, using all the batter.

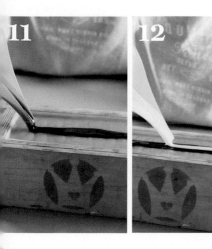 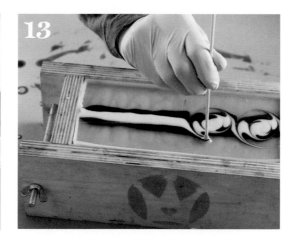

1. Pour the remaining blue batter in a wide line own the middle of the yellow soap.

2. Pour a thin line of white down the middle of he blue line, leaving a line of blue on either side.

13. Insert a chopstick about a ¼ inch deep into the white line, about an inch from the end of the mold. Swirl the chopstick in a spiral pattern from the white line, to just inside the blue lines. Lift the chopstick out of the soap, wipe the excess soap off, and repeat the process, making spirals in the rest of the soap.

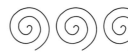

FINAL STEPS

4. Spritz the top of the soap with 99% rubbing cohol to help prevent soda ash.

5. Allow the soap to set for at least 4 to 5 days efore attempting to unmold. This recipe utilizes any soft oils, so it takes longer than usual to et. If the soap is difficult to remove from the er, allow it to set for another 24 hours before tempting to unmold again.

16. Once the soap is removed from the liner, turn it sideways to cut into bars to avoid dragging the blue and white lines through the yellow. Allow the bars to cure in a well-ventilated area for 4 to 6 weeks before using, turning them every few days to ensure that they cure evenly.

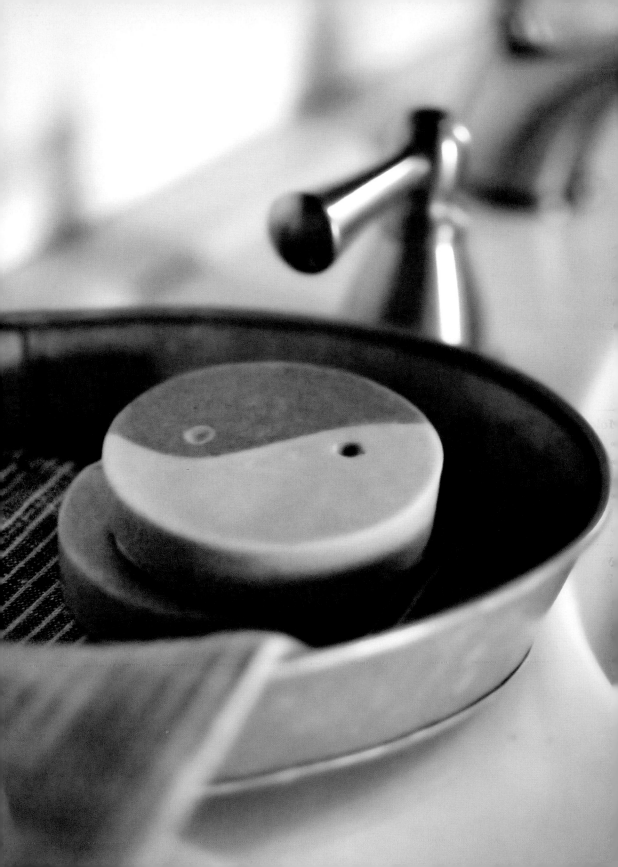

White & Red

WINE YIN/YANG

Makes 12 bars

This unique soap style will get noticed. In Chinese philosophy, the concept of yin and yang is that opposite forces complement one another. This soap is a good example of that. The white and red wines work together to create beautiful black and pink hues in a nourishing bar that is full of antioxidants.

STAGE 1: MAKE THE MAIN SOAPS

WHITE WINE RECIPE

Mold and Special Tools

» 12-bar round silicone mold

» 2 manila folders to make the dividers

» 12 plastic drinking straws, cut in half

› Tape

Lye-Water Amounts

2.3 ounces lye (7% superfat)

8 ounces white wine (2.8 ounces reduced, per instructions)

2.8 ounces distilled water

1 teaspoon sodium lactate (optional)

Oil Amounts

2.6 ounces palm oil (15%)

3.4 ounces coconut oil (20%)

0.9 ounce meadowfoam oil (5%)

1.7 ounces sesame oil (10%)

2.6 ounces rice bran oil (15%)

6 ounces olive oil pure (35%)

Essential Oil

0.7 ounce lavender 40/42*

Colorants

1 teaspoon rose clay dispersed into 1 tablespoon distilled water

1 teaspoon activated charcoal dispersed into 1 tablespoon meadowfoam oil

Regular lavender essential oil will work, but this variety has been specifically blended to last in cold-process soap.

Note: The wine must be prepared ahead of time, and the soap requires two days to make, so allow extra time for this recipe. This is a two-person design — you will need a buddy to hold down the dividers while you pour the soap.

Safe Soaping!

Wear proper safety gear the whole time.

Work in a well-ventilated space.

No distractions (keep kids and pets away).

RED WINE RECIPE

Lye-Water Amounts

2.3 ounces lye (7% superfat)

8 ounces red wine (2.8 ounces reduced, per instructions)

2.8 ounces distilled water

1 teaspoon sodium lactate (optional)

Oil Amounts

2.6 ounces palm oil (15%)

3.4 ounces coconut oil (20%)

0.9 ounce meadowfoam oil (5%)

1.7 ounces sesame oil (10%)

2.6 ounces rice bran oil (15%)

6 ounces olive oil pure (35%)

Essential Oil

0.7 ounce black pepper essential oil

PREPARE THE MOLD

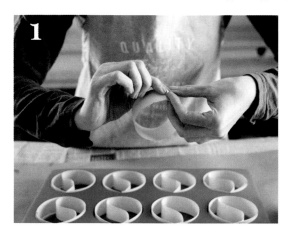

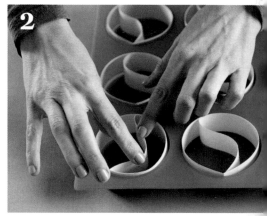

Place the mold on a cutting board. Cut the manila file folders into 12 strips, each 1 1/2 inches wide and 17 inches long. Make sure the cuts are straight, otherwise the soap will leak under the dividers. Repeat the following steps for each individual cavity:

1. Fold the strip in half. Wrap the strip around the inside circumference of one of the round cavities. There will be a little bit of overlap.

2. Grasp the inner layer of the paper, about 1 inch down from the folded end. Pull only that layer to the center of the mold. This should create the signature swirl of the yin/yang symbol.

3. Once you have a good yin/yang shape, carefully pinch each divider to remove it from mold, and secure the shape with tape. Place the divider back in the mold.

PREPARE THE WINES

Before using wine in soap, you must remove as much of the alcohol as possible. For each wine, pour 8 ounces into a small saucepan (do not combine them) and bring to a boil. Reduce the heat and allow the wine to simmer for 5 to 10 minutes. Remove the wines from the heat and place them in an ice bath or the fridge to cool to around 60°F (15.5 °C).

MAKE THE SOAP MIXTURE

1. Measure 2.8 ounces of the cooled, boiled white wine into a heat-safe container. Add 2.8 ounces of distilled water to the white wine. Slowly add the lye to the water-wine mixture (never the other way around), adding a little bit of lye at a time, and stir until each addition is dissolved. There is a strong, unpleasant smell that comes from mixing the lye with the wine, but it will fade in the soap, and is completely normal. Set the lye mixture aside until it cools to under 130°F (54°C). If using sodium lactate, add it to the lye-water and stir to combine.

2. Melt the palm oil and coconut oil in their original containers, and measure the melted oils into a bowl large enough to hold all of the batter with room for mixing. Measure the meadowfoam oil, sesame oil, rice bran oil, and olive oil pure into the container. If the oils go cloudy, microwave

in 15-second bursts, stirring between each time. Try to keep the temperatures of both batches of oils within five degrees of each other for best results.

3. Repeat steps 1 and 2 with the recipe for red wine. At the end of this step, you should have a red wine-lye mixture, a white wine-lye mixture, and two separate containers of oils.

4. When the oils and the lye mixtures are all under 120°F (49°C), slowly add the red wine-lye mixture to one container of oils, and the white wine-lye mixture to the other container of oils. Tap the stick blender a few times on the bottom of the bowl to release any bubbles. *Do not turn on the stick blender until it is fully immersed.* Stick-blend the white wine batter first for 10 seconds. Next, stick-blend the red wine batter for 10 seconds. They should both be at a thin trace.

COLOR AND POUR

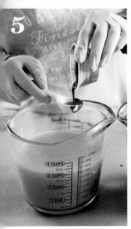
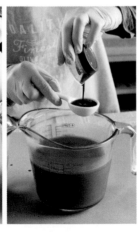
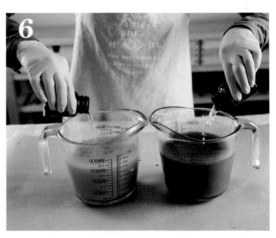

5. To the white wine soap, add 1½ teaspoons of the rose clay dispersion.
To the red wine soap, add 1 tablespoon of the activated charcoal dispersion.

6. Add the lavender essential oil to the white wine soap and the black pepper essential oil to the red wine soap. Whisk the lighter soap first to incorporate the colorant and essential oil, then use the same whisk to mix the darker soap.

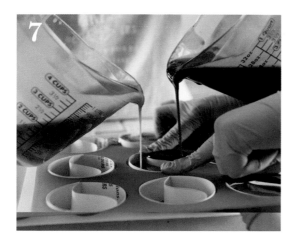

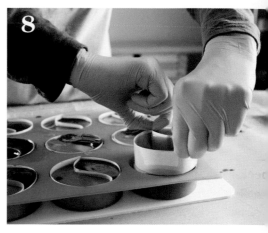

7. Have your buddy firmly press the paper dividers against the bottom of the mold while you carefully pour the black and pink soap batter at the same time into one cavity, black on one side of the divider, pink on the other. Keep the levels of the black and pink even. Repeat this process until all of the cavities are filled.

8. Remove the dividers very carefully. Pinch the divider at either end of the center divider, and quickly and carefully pull it straight up and out of the soap, right into the trash can. Repeat this process for each soap.

Safety note: Carefully watch how full you are filling the molds, remembering that the dividers are deeper than the mold itself. If you pour them too full, the soap will spill out when the divider is removed

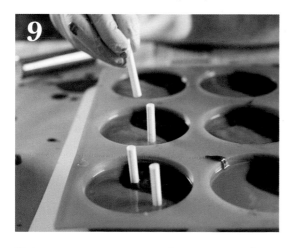

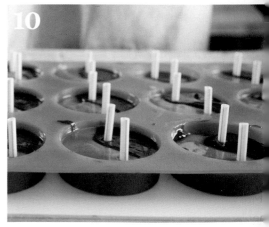

9. Insert two straws into each soap: one in the center of the bulge in the pink side, and one centered in the bulge in the black side.

10. Allow the soap to set for 24 hours before removing the straws.

Carefully remove the straws by twisting them, then pulling straight up and out of the soap. If the raw pulls out without taking the plug of soap inside with it, use a small chopstick or similar-sized ol to pull out the circle of soap. Do not remove the bars from the mold, or the "filling" soap will seep der the main soap.

FILL IN THE DOTS

Special Tools

- Mini mixer
- 2 droppers
- Spare mold that holds at least 6 ounces

Lye-Water Amounts

- 0.6 ounce lye
- 1.3 ounces distilled water

Oil Amount

- 4 ounces coconut oil

Colorants

- 1/4 teaspoon rose clay dispersed into 3/4 teaspoon water
- 1/4 teaspoon activated charcoal dispersed into 3/4 teaspoon olive oil pure

MAKE THE SOAP MIXTURE

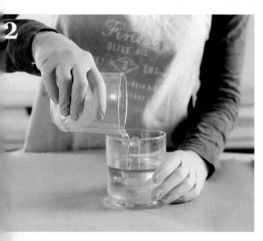

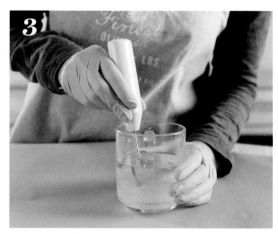

Slowly and carefully add the lye to the water ver the other way around) and stir until all of lye is dissolved. Set aside to cool.

Measure and melt the coconut oil in a con- er large enough to hold both the oil and the mixture with room to stir. Using a tall, narrow tainer makes it easier to mix such a small ount of soap.

3. When the oil is between 90° and 95°F (32–35°C) and the lye-water is between 130° and 135°F (54–57°C), slowly and carefully add the lye-water to the oil. Stir with a mini mixer or a stick blender until it reaches trace. The recipes uses 100 percent coconut oil to ensure that it will trace quickly.

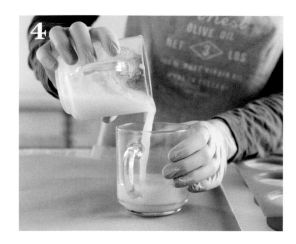

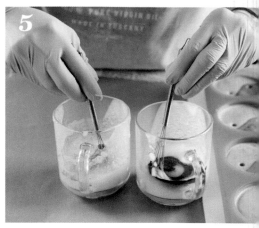

4. Once the soap has reached trace, divide the batter in half and add the colorants.

5. To one container, add ½ teaspoon of the ro[s] clay dispersion; to the other, add ½ teaspoon o[f] the activated charcoal dispersion. Stir each col[or] in well.

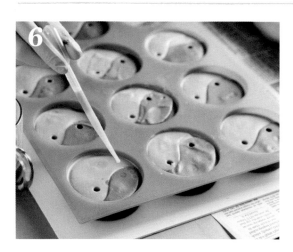

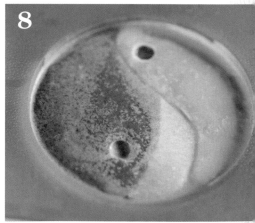

6. Using a dropper, fill up the holes in the yin/yang soaps using opposite colors: pink soap batter in the black soap, and black soap batter in the pink soap.

7. Pour any excess batter into the extra mold.

8. Allow the soaps to set for 48 hours before attempting to unmold. Allow the bars to cure i[n] a well-ventilated area for 4 to 6 weeks before using, turning them every few days to ensure that they cure evenly.

Resources

General Supplies

Bramble Berry, Inc.
877-627-7883
www.brambleberry.com

From Nature with Love
800-520-2060
www.fromnaturewithlove.com

Frontier Natural Products Co-op
800-669-3275
www.frontiercoop.com

GloryBee Foods
800-456-7923
http://naturalcrafts.glorybee.com

Hoegger Goat Supply
800-221-4628
http://hoeggerfarmyard.com

Liberty Natural Products, Inc.
800-289-8427
www.libertynatural.com

Majestic Mountain Sage
435-755-0863
www.thesage.com

Mountain Rose Herbs
800-879-3337
www.mountainroseherbs.com

San Francisco Herb Co.
800-227-4530
www.sfherb.com

Summers Past Farms
800-390-1523
www.summerspastfarms.com

Wild Weeds
800-839-4101
www.wildweeds.com

Essential Oils, Fragrance Oils & Colorants

Bramble Berry, Inc.
877-627-7883
www.brambleberry.com

From Nature with Love
800-520-2060
www.fromnaturewithlove.com

The Perfumery
502-498-8804
http://theperfumery.com

Rainbow Meadow, Inc.
517-764-9765
www.rainbowmeadow.com

SoapGoods
404-924-9080
www.soapgoods.com

Wholesale Supplies Plus, Inc.
800-359-0944
www.wholesalesuppliesplus.com

Oils & Fats

Bramble Berry, Inc.
877-627-7883
www.brambleberry.com

Columbus Foods
800-322-6457
www.soaperschoice.com

Hoegger Goat Supply
800-221-4628
http://hoeggerfarmyard.com

Oils of Aloha
800-367-6010
www.oilsofaloha.com

Spectrum Chemical Manufacturing Corp.
800-813-1514
www.spectrumchemical.com

Welch, Holme & Clark Co. Inc.
973-465-1200
www.welch-holme-clark.com

Essential Oil Purity Testing

Spectrix Labs
831-427-9336
http://spectrixlab.com

Tutorials

Soap Queen
www.soapqueen.com

Videos

Soap Queen TV YouTube
www.youtube.com/user/soapqueentv

Index

Personalize Your Personal Care with More DIY Books from Storey

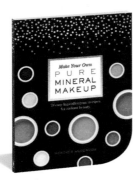

by Heather Anderson

Making naturally derived cosmetics is easy — and inexpensive! These 79 recipes for eye shadow, foundation, concealer, blush, and more protect and promote healthy skin, while detailed directions show how to customize for your skin type and color.

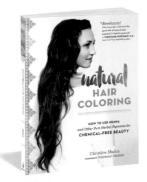

by Christine Shahin

Achieve rich, natural-looking shades of brown, black, red, and even blond by combining henna with three other plant pigments. This accessible guide shows you how to get a variety of stunning hair colors without any chemicals.

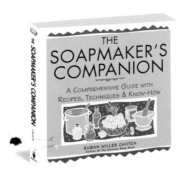

by Susan Miller Cavitch

Craft vegetable-based and transparent soaps with a range of special design features. This comprehensive resource for beginner and advanced soapmakers alike includes 40 recipes and covers the chemistry of soapmaking and business basics.

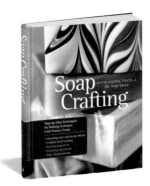

by Anne-Marie Faiola

Making soap is easy! This one stop resource for soapmakers of all skill levels includes 31 recipes and step-by-step instructions. Explore the full range of special effects, colors, additives, and molds available.

Join the conversation. Share your experience with this book, learn more about Storey Publishing's authors, and read original essays and book excerpts at storey.com. Look for our books wherever quality books are sold or call 800-441-5700.